ABOUT THE AUTHOR

Wendy D. Palmer

Wendy D. Palmer is an independent author and a retired registered nurse and medical case manager with over three decades of experience in trauma, emergency, acute care, and interventional radiology nursing. Wendy has lived with Young-Onset Parkinson's Disease for over 20 years and has devoted much time into research regarding brain health. She is always on the lookout for solutions to health problems. With Parkinson's disease, she has had many health challenges to find solutions for: chronic fatigue, brain fog, and insomnia. Wendy explores themes of spirituality, longevity, health, nutrition, grief, and caregiving. Her work blends professional insight with personal wisdom to support readers facing loss and health challenges.

ABSTRACT

Discover the revolutionary potential of methylene blue, a century-old compound with modern applications for optimal health. This comprehensive guide explores how this remarkable substance can enhance cellular energy, boost cognitive function, and support overall well-being. Drawing from both scientific research and practical experience, we'll explore ten powerful ways this versatile compound can transform your health, along with detailed protocols for safe and effective use. Whether you're seeking to improve mental clarity, increase energy levels, or support your body's natural healing processes, this book provides the knowledge and practical guidance you need to harness the full potential of methylene blue.

TABLE OF CONTENTS

INTRODUCTION

In a world where health optimization has become increasingly complex, the search for effective, scientifically backed solutions has led many to overlook one of the most remarkable therapeutic compounds available: methylene blue. As a registered nurse with over three decades of experience and someone who has extensively studied cellular health while managing Young-Onset Parkinson's Disease, I've discovered that this powerful molecule offers unprecedented potential for enhancing human health and vitality.

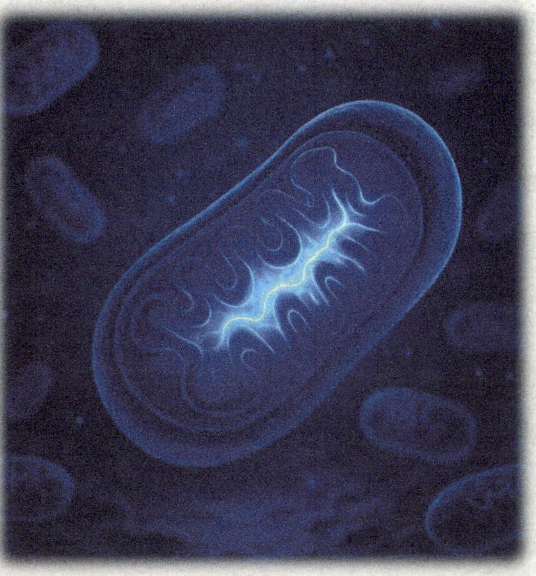

Methylene blue's journey from laboratory curiosity to therapeutic powerhouse represents one of the most fascinating chapters in medical science. This remarkable compound works at the cellular level, enhancing mitochondrial function and promoting optimal energy production in ways that conventional treatments often cannot achieve. Its applications span from supporting cognitive function to enhancing cellular repair mechanisms, making it a versatile tool in the pursuit of optimal health.

In this comprehensive guide, we'll explore the science behind methylene blue's therapeutic potential, delving into its mechanisms of action while maintaining accessibility for both healthcare professionals and enthusiasts alike. This book aims to bridge the gap between complex biochemistry and practical application, providing you with the knowledge and protocols necessary to harness the benefits of methylene blue safely and effectively.

From understanding proper dosing protocols to exploring potential interactions with medications, we'll address critical questions about safety, efficacy, and optimal usage. We'll examine the latest research findings and translate them into actionable insights, ensuring you have the tools needed to make informed decisions about incorporating methylene blue into your health regimen.

As we explore the ten transformative benefits of methylene blue, you'll discover how this compound can support everything from brain health to cellular regeneration. We'll delve into practical considerations for storage, quality

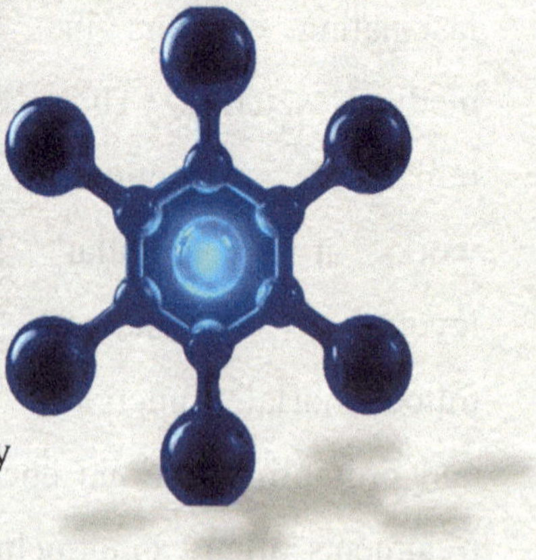

assessment, and long-term usage while maintaining a focus on safety and evidence-based recommendations.

My goal in writing this book is to provide you with a thorough understanding of methylene blue's potential, while emphasizing the importance of informed and careful usage. Whether you're a healthcare professional seeking to expand your therapeutic toolkit or an individual interested in optimizing your health, this guide will serve as your comprehensive resource for understanding and implementing methylene blue therapy effectively and safely.

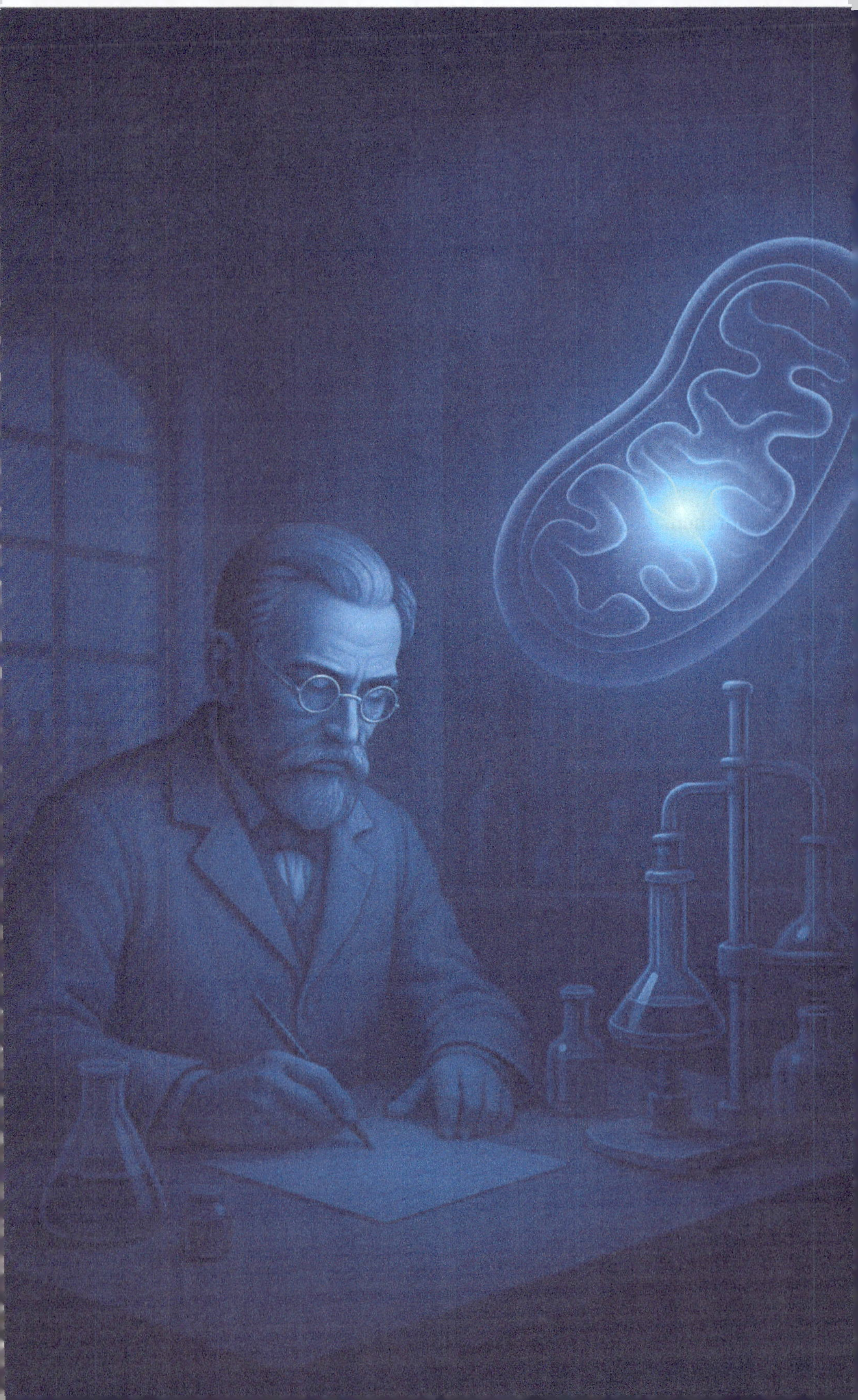

CHAPTER 1

UNDERSTANDING THE BLUE REVOLUTION: THE SCIENCE AND HISTORY OF METHYLENE BLUE

In the bustling laboratory of a German chemist in 1876, an accidental discovery would forever change the course of medical history. What began as a quest to create synthetic indigo dye would lead to the revelation of methylene blue, a compound that would prove to be far more valuable to humanity than anyone could have imagined. This serendipitous discovery would launch decades of scientific investigation into the remarkable properties and therapeutic potential of methylene blue. As a registered nurse who has witnessed the evolution of medical treatments over three decades, I've seen firsthand how certain compounds can revolutionize our approach to health and healing. Methylene blue stands out as one of the most versatile and fascinating molecules in modern medicine.

The journey of understanding methylene blue reveals a compound that operates at the very foundation of cellular function. Its unique molecular structure allows it to penetrate cell membranes and interact with our mitochondria—the powerhouses of our cells—in ways that enhance energy production and cellular efficiency. This fundamental interaction forms the basis for its wide-ranging therapeutic applications, from treating malaria in its early days to its current use in modern medical procedures and emerging therapeutic protocols.

In this chapter, we'll explore the core mechanisms that make methylene blue such a powerful therapeutic agent. We'll examine its basic chemistry, how it interacts with cellular processes, and the scientific principles that explain its remarkable effects on human health. Understanding these foundations is crucial for anyone looking to harness the full potential of this compound safely and effectively.

Exploring the science and history of methylene blue reveals why this compound has captivated researchers and healthcare practitioners worldwide. Its ability to enhance cellular energy, combat oxidative stress, and strengthen key biological processes makes it a powerful ally in the pursuit of optimal health. Whether you're a clinician expanding your therapeutic toolkit or an individual seeking advanced wellness solutions, understanding the core principles of methylene blue will provide practical insights for real-world application.

The Accidental Discovery: From Textile Dye to Medical Marvel

In 1876, German chemist Heinrich Caro made a groundbreaking discovery while working at BASF, though he couldn't have known the profound impact it would have on modern medicine. While attempting to synthesize artificial indigo dye for the textile industry, Caro created methylene blue - a vivid blue compound that would become the first fully synthetic drug used in medicine[1 2 3]. This serendipitous creation marked the beginning of a scientific revolution that would transform our understanding of cellular biology and therapeutic interventions.

The transition of methylene blue from an industrial dye to a medical breakthrough began when scientists noticed its remarkable ability to stain cells selectively and microorganisms[2 3 5]. This property caught the attention of pioneering researchers, such as Paul Ehrlich, who recognized that methylene blue's staining capabilities might indicate therapeutic potential. In 1887, Polish pathologist Czeslaw Checinski discovered that methylene blue could effectively stain malaria parasites[2], leading to a crucial breakthrough in the visualization and study of these deadly pathogens.

Paul Ehrlich and Paul Guttmann's subsequent work in 1891 established methylene blue as the first synthetic pharmaceutical when they successfully used it to treat malaria patients[1 2 3 5]. This achievement was particularly significant because, unlike natural remedies such as quinine extracted from cinchona bark, methylene blue could be manufactured consistently and at scale, laying the groundwork for modern pharmaceutical production[2].

The compound's versatility soon became apparent as researchers uncovered multiple medical applications. In 1933, scientist Matilda Brooks discovered the effectiveness of methylene blue as an antidote for carbon monoxide and cyanide poisoning1. The compound also revolutionized laboratory diagnostics through its role in the development of the Giemsa stain for blood cell analysis[3]. It became instrumental in testing milk quality by detecting bacterial contamination[4].

Methylene blue's unique molecular structure allows it to cross the blood-brain barrier and interact with cellular processes in ways that continue to intrigue researchers today. Its ability to enhance mitochondrial function and reduce oxidative stress has led to investigations into its potential for treating neurodegenerative disorders, psychiatric conditions, and various other medical applications[5]. The compound's ability to carry electrons makes it particularly effective in supporting cellular energy production. This property underlies many of its therapeutic benefits.

The evolution of methylene blue from textile dye to therapeutic agent exemplifies how careful scientific observation and methodical investigation can reveal unexpected medical applications. While initially valued for its color-fast properties in fabric, methylene blue's ability to interact with biological systems at the cellular level has established it as a versatile tool in modern medicine. Its development also paved the way for synthetic drug research, inspiring the creation of numerous other therapeutic compounds, including modern antimalarial medications like chloroquine[2].

Today, methylene blue continues to be studied for its diverse therapeutic applications, from its traditional use in emergency medicine to emerging research in neuroscience and cellular health[5]. It's a remarkable journey from accidental discovery to medical marvel, demonstrating the often unexpected paths through which scientific breakthroughs can emerge. As research continues, new applications for this versatile compound are being discovered, further enhancing its already impressive legacy in the field of medical science.

Understanding Methylene Blue's Molecular Structure

To truly understand the remarkable capabilities of methylene blue, we must first examine its unique molecular structure. This foundation enables its diverse therapeutic applications. At its core, methylene blue is a heterocyclic aromatic compound with the chemical formula $C_{16}H_{18}ClN_3S$[6 7 8]. This seemingly complex arrangement of atoms creates a molecule that possesses extraordinary biological properties and therapeutic potential.

The backbone of methylene blue consists of a phenothiazine core - a tricyclic structure containing both sulfur and nitrogen atoms within its rings[1 7 10]. This core is enhanced by two dimethylamino groups positioned at specific points on the molecule, along with a chloride counterion[1 7 9]. While this might sound technical, this precise architectural arrangement is what allows methylene blue to perform its cellular magic. The molecule's structure enables it to easily cross cell membranes and interact with various biological systems, particularly our cellular energy factories—the mitochondria.

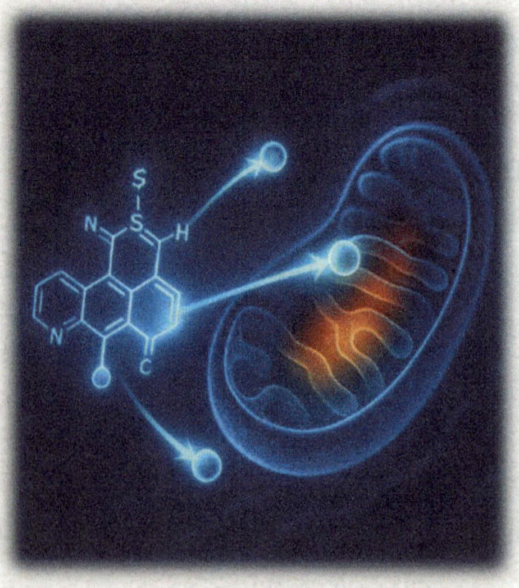

One of methylene blue's most fascinating structural features is its ability to act as a redox agent, meaning it can efficiently accept and donate electrons. In its oxidized form, methylene blue appears as the characteristic deep blue color with which we're familiar. However, when it accepts electrons, it transforms into its reduced form, known as leucomethylene blue, which is colorless[1 7]. This color change isn't just a chemical curiosity - it's a visual indicator of the molecule's ability to participate in crucial cellular energy processes.

The molecular design of methylene blue makes it highly soluble in water while maintaining the ability to pass through lipid-based cell membranes8. This dual nature is crucial for its therapeutic applications, as it allows the compound to be easily absorbed and distributed throughout the body. When dissolved in water, methylene blue forms a deep blue solution, though in its pure form, it actually appears as a dark green crystalline powder[7 8].

Perhaps most remarkably, methylene blue's structure allows it to serve as an electron shuttle in biological systems. Its molecular arrangement enables it to accept electrons from compounds like NADH and $FADH_2$[1], and then transfer these electrons to other molecules within the cell. This electron-carrying capability is fundamental to its role in enhancing mitochondrial function and cellular energy production.

The size and shape of the methylene blue molecule are also perfectly suited for its therapeutic roles. With a molecular weight of 319.85 g/mol6 [8], it's small enough to cross the blood-brain barrier efficiently. This crucial feature enables its cognitive and neuroprotective effects. This characteristic, combined with its ability to interact with cellular components, makes it an effective compound for various therapeutic applications.

Understanding the molecular structure of methylene blue helps explain its remarkable versatility in medical applications. The compound's ability to readily change between its oxidized and reduced states, coupled with its optimal size and solubility properties, creates a powerful therapeutic tool. These structural characteristics enable methylene blue to function effectively as an antioxidant, energy enhancer, and cellular protector[8 9].

The molecular architecture of methylene blue also explains its stability and extended shelf life when stored properly. The compound's structure remains stable under normal conditions, though it can be sensitive to light exposure. This stability, combined with its solubility properties[8], makes it practical for both clinical and personal use when appropriate storage guidelines are followed.

Basic Chemistry and Properties of Methylene Blue

The remarkable therapeutic potential of methylene blue stems from its unique chemical composition and properties. At its most basic level, methylene blue is a synthetic compound with the chemical formula $C_{16}H_{18}ClN_3S$[11 7 8 13], consisting of a phenothiazine core structure enhanced by specific molecular groups that give it its characteristic properties and therapeutic capabilities[11 1 7 9].

In its pure form, methylene blue appears as a dark green crystalline powder, but it transforms into its familiar deep blue color when dissolved in water[1 7]. This color-changing property isn't merely cosmetic, it's a visual indicator of the compound's remarkable ability to participate in redox reactions, switching between its oxidized blue form and reduced colorless form (leucomethylene blue)[1 12]. This unique characteristic makes methylene blue an exceptional electron carrier in biological systems.

One of methylene blue's most significant properties is its high water solubility combined with its ability to cross lipid-based cell membranes. When dissolved in water, it forms a slightly acidic solution with a pH of approximately 6 at standard concentrations[11]. This dual nature being both water-soluble and able to penetrate cellular barriers is crucial for its therapeutic effectiveness, allowing it to be easily absorbed and distributed throughout the body.

The molecular structure of methylene blue comprises three fused rings that form its phenothiazine core, along with dimethylamino groups and a chloride counterion[11 1 7 9]. This precise architectural arrangement gives the compound its relatively small molecular mass of 319.85 g/mol[11 8], enabling it to readily cross the blood-brain barrier, a critical feature for its cognitive and neuroprotective applications.

Methylene blue exhibits specific light absorption characteristics, with maximum absorption occurring between 664 and 670 nanometers in solution[1 7]. This property not only contributes to its deep blue color but also makes it useful in various diagnostic and therapeutic applications. The compound's photoactive nature means it responds to light in ways that can be harnessed for certain medical treatments[7].

Perhaps most importantly for therapeutic applications, methylene blue functions as a reversible redox indicator with a redox midpoint potential of +0.01 V1. This property enables it to efficiently accept electrons from compounds such as NADH and $FADH_2$, and then transfer these electrons to other molecules within cellular systems. This electron-shuttling capability is fundamental to its role in enhancing mitochondrial function and cellular energy production.

The stability of methylene blue under normal conditions makes it practical for clinical use; however, it requires proper storage, away from light exposure, to maintain its efficacy. When exposed to reducing agents, such as glucose in the presence of sodium hydroxide, methylene blue undergoes its characteristic color change, demonstrating its redox cycling capabilities[1].

Understanding these basic chemical properties helps explain the diverse therapeutic applications of methylene blue. Its ability to participate in cellular redox reactions, cross biological barriers, and interact with various cellular components makes it a versatile compound in medical applications. From treating methemoglobinemia by converting ferric iron in hemoglobin to its ferrous state[11 8], to its potential applications in neurodegenerative disorders, these fundamental properties underlie its therapeutic potential.

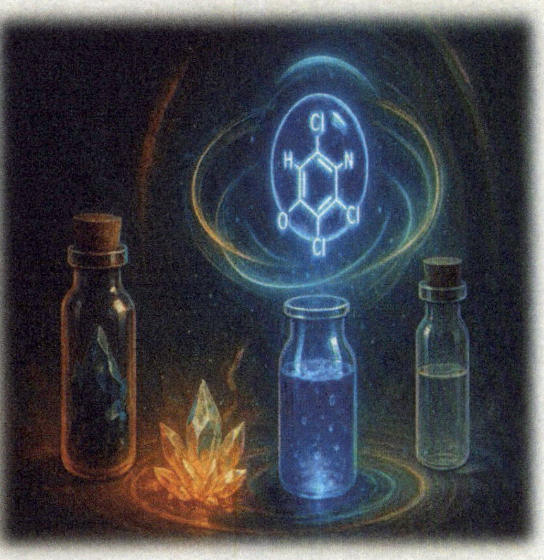

The compound's interaction with biological systems extends beyond its redox capabilities. Methylene blue can inhibit certain enzymatic processes, particularly those mediated by cyclic GMP, and has demonstrated the ability to prevent tau protein aggregation, a process implicated in various neurodegenerative conditions[7,9]. Its antioxidant properties, combined with its ability to enhance mitochondrial function, make it a powerful tool for cellular protection and energy enhancement.

When working with methylene blue, it's crucial to understand that its concentration can affect its behavior in solution. At higher concentrations, the molecules can form dimers and aggregates, which may influence their therapeutic effectiveness[1]. This property necessitates careful attention to proper dosing and administration protocols to achieve optimal results.

Early Medical Applications and Breakthrough Discoveries

The evolution of methylene blue from industrial dye to groundbreaking therapeutic agent represents one of medicine's most remarkable transformations. In 1891, German physician Paul Ehrlich and his colleague Paul Guttmann achieved a historic milestone by successfully using methylene blue to treat malaria patients[1 14 16 17], establishing it as the first fully synthetic drug in medical history[1 17]. This breakthrough marked the beginning of a new era in pharmaceutical development, shifting the focus from traditional plant and animal-derived remedies to laboratory-created medicines.

The compound's early medical applications were diverse and groundbreaking. Its ability to selectively stain and target Plasmodium parasites made it an effective antimalarial treatment[16], while its strong staining properties revolutionized microscopy and surgical procedures. Robert Koch utilized methylene blue's staining capabilities to visualize bacteria under the microscope as early as 1880[15], advancing our understanding of microbiology. In surgical settings, the compound proved invaluable for mapping lymph nodes and enhancing procedural precision[14 17].

A significant advancement occurred in 1933 when scientist Matilda Brooks discovered the effectiveness of methylene blue as an antidote for carbon monoxide and cyanide poisoning[1]. This discovery expanded the compound's life-saving potential in emergency medicine. Additionally, methylene blue became the standard treatment for methemoglobinemia, a potentially life-threatening blood disorder that affects oxygen transport[18]. Its ability to convert methemoglobin back to functional hemoglobin remains an FDA-approved application today[18].

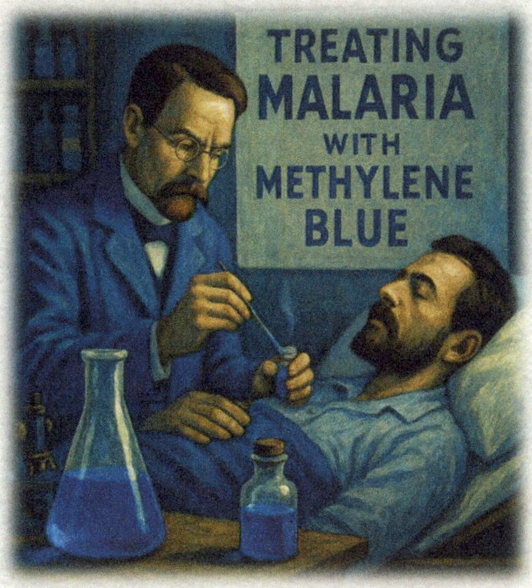

Methylene blue's influence extends far beyond its direct applications. The compound served as a prototype for developing numerous modern pharmaceuticals, including antimalarial drugs like chloroquine, antihistamines, and antipsychotic medications such as chlorpromazine[1]. Its success inspired researchers to explore synthetic solutions to medical challenges and design drugs targeting specific biological pathways[1 16].

The compound's antimicrobial properties were recognized long before the advent of antibiotics, making it a valuable tool in treating various bacterial and protozoal infections[14]. Its unique ability to cross the blood-brain barrier and interact with cellular processes sparked investigations into potential applications for neurological conditions. This versatility in medical applications stems from methylene blue's fundamental properties, its ability to participate in redox reactions, penetrate cellular membranes, and enhance mitochondrial function.

In modern medicine, methylene blue continues to demonstrate its versatility. Its application in photodynamic therapy has shown promise in treating certain cancers, while its potential neuroprotective properties are being investigated for various neurodegenerative conditions. The compound's role in enhancing mitochondrial function and reducing oxidative stress has led to research into its possible benefits for cognitive enhancement and cellular energy production.

The scientific understanding of methylene blue's mechanisms has evolved significantly since its first medical applications. Research has revealed its ability to inhibit nitric oxide synthase, modulate the electron transport chain, and prevent tau protein aggregation—processes implicated in various pathological conditions. These discoveries continue to expand our understanding of the compound's therapeutic potential.

Methylene blue's journey from dye to therapeutic agent exemplifies the importance of scientific observation and methodical investigation in medical advancement. Its development as the first synthetic drug laid the groundwork for modern pharmaceutical research and production methods[1 17]. Today, it remains a valuable tool in medical practice, with applications ranging from emergency medicine to emerging therapeutic protocols in neuroscience and cellular health.

The compound's safety profile, established through decades of clinical use, along with its well-understood mechanisms of action, makes it a reliable option in various medical contexts. However, proper dosing, administration protocols, and consideration of potential interactions remain crucial for the effective therapeutic use of this medication. As research continues, new applications for this versatile compound are being discovered, further enhancing its already impressive legacy in the field of medical science.

The Evolution of Methylene Blue in Modern Medicine

The modern medical landscape has witnessed a remarkable evolution in the understanding and application of methylene blue, transforming it from its historical roots into a sophisticated therapeutic tool[5 14 19]. This progression represents one of medicine's most fascinating journeys of drug development and application, demonstrating how scientific innovation can unlock new potential in existing compounds.

In contemporary medicine, methylene blue has found numerous FDA-approved applications, with the treatment of methemoglobinemia being its primary indicated use[18]. The compound's ability to restore normal oxygen-carrying capacity to blood by converting methemoglobin back to functional hemoglobin has made it an indispensable tool in emergency medicine[18]. This application exemplifies the compound's fundamental mechanism of action - its capacity to participate in critical electron transfer processes within biological systems[5 18].

The research landscape surrounding methylene blue has undergone significant expansion in recent decades. Scientists have uncovered its potential in treating various conditions, from its use in photodynamic therapy for certain cancers to its application in managing vasodilatory shock[19]. Its ability to cross the blood-brain barrier has sparked particular interest in neuroscience, where researchers are investigating its potential for treating neurodegenerative disorders and enhancing cognitive function[5].

One of the most significant modern developments has been the understanding of methylene blue's role in mitochondrial function. Research has revealed its ability to enhance cellular energy production by improving the efficiency of the electron transport efficiency[5]. This discovery has led to investigations into its potential for treating conditions characterized by mitochondrial dysfunction, including various neurological disorders and age-related cognitive decline[5].

In surgical applications, methylene blue remains invaluable for tissue staining and mapping procedures. Its use in sentinel lymph node mapping for cancer surgery has become standard practice in many institutions[14 19],

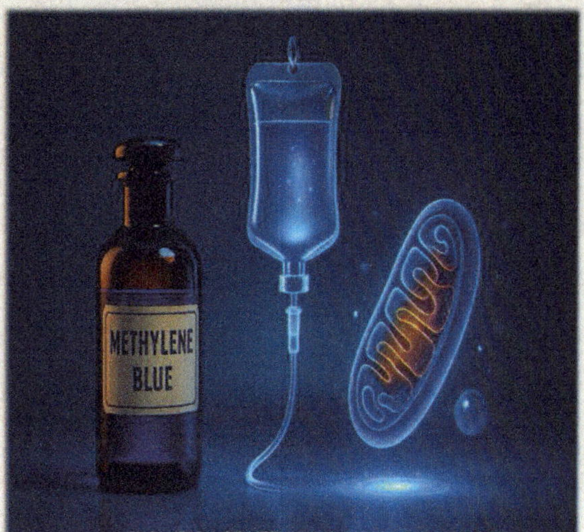

EVOLUTION OF METHYLENE IN MODERN MEDICINE

demonstrating how its original staining properties continue to find new medical applications[5 19 18]. The compound's ability to selectively target certain tissues has also led to its investigation in novel diagnostic techniques[16 14 19].

The antimicrobial properties of methylene blue have gained renewed attention in the era of antibiotic resistance. Research has shown its effectiveness against various pathogens, and its potential as an adjunct therapy in treating resistant infections is being explored[14]. Additionally, its antiviral properties have sparked interest in its potential role in managing viral infections[14].

Modern pharmaceutical research has also focused on optimizing the delivery systems and formulations of methylene blue. Scientists are developing new ways to enhance its bioavailability and targeting capabilities, potentially expanding its therapeutic applications. These developments include novel encapsulation methods and combination therapies that may improve its efficacy in various medical contexts.

The compound's safety profile has been extensively studied in modern medicine, resulting in a deeper understanding of its contraindications and potential interactions. This research has helped establish clear guidelines for its use in different medical scenarios, making it safer and more effective for both traditional and emerging applications.

Perhaps most intriguingly, methylene blue's role in cellular energy production has led to investigations into its potential anti-aging properties. Research suggests it may help protect against cellular damage and support healthy aging through its antioxidant properties and ability to enhance mitochondrial function[5]. This area represents one of the most promising frontiers in methylene blue research.

The evolution of methylene blue in modern medicine continues to unfold as new research reveals additional therapeutic applications. Its journey from a simple dye to a versatile medical compound underscores the importance of continued scientific investigation into established substances. As our understanding of cellular processes deepens, methylene blue's unique properties position it as a valuable tool in addressing various medical challenges, from acute emergencies to chronic conditions affecting cellular energy metabolism[5,18].

How Methylene Blue Interacts with Human Biology

At the cellular level, methylene blue operates as a remarkable biological multitool, interacting with various systems in ways that can profoundly impact human health. This versatile compound's primary mechanism of action centers on its unique ability to serve as an electron carrier within our cells, particularly in the mitochondria—our cellular powerhouses[20]. By facilitating electron transport and enhancing energy production, methylene blue helps optimize cellular function across multiple body systems.

The foundation of methylene blue's biological interaction lies in its molecular structure, which allows it to cross both cell membranes and the blood-brain barrier easily[18]. Once inside cells, it participates in critical redox reactions, meaning it can both accept and donate electrons[20]. This property makes it particularly valuable in supporting mitochondrial function, where it helps maintain efficient energy production even when natural cellular processes are compromised.

In mitochondria, methylene blue acts as an alternative electron carrier in the electron transport chain (ETC). When parts of this vital energy-producing system become damaged or inefficient, methylene blue can bypass these problematic areas, helping to maintain ATP production—the cellular energy currency[20]. This process not only supports energy production but also reduces the formation of harmful reactive oxygen species (ROS), which can damage cellular components[20].

One of methylene blue's most significant interactions occurs in red blood cells, where it plays a crucial role in maintaining proper oxygen transport. In cases of methemoglobinemia - a condition where hemoglobin becomes oxidized and unable to carry oxygen effectively - methylene blue converts to its reduced form (leucomethylene blue) within red blood cells[21 22 24]. This reduced form then converts the dysfunctional ferric iron (Fe^{3+}) in hemoglobin back to its oxygen-carrying ferrous state (Fe^{2+}), restoring normal oxygen delivery to tissues[21 18].

The compound's interaction with enzyme systems represents another crucial aspect of its biological activity. Methylene blue inhibits several important enzymes, including nitric oxide synthase (NOS) and guanylate cyclase[21 22 26]. This inhibition affects vascular tone and can be particularly beneficial in managing certain cardiovascular conditions. However, it's important to note that this same mechanism requires careful consideration when using methylene blue alongside certain medications, particularly those affecting serotonin levels[23 25].

In the brain, methylene blue's interactions are particularly fascinating. Its ability to cross the blood-brain barrier allows it to support neuronal energy production directly[20].

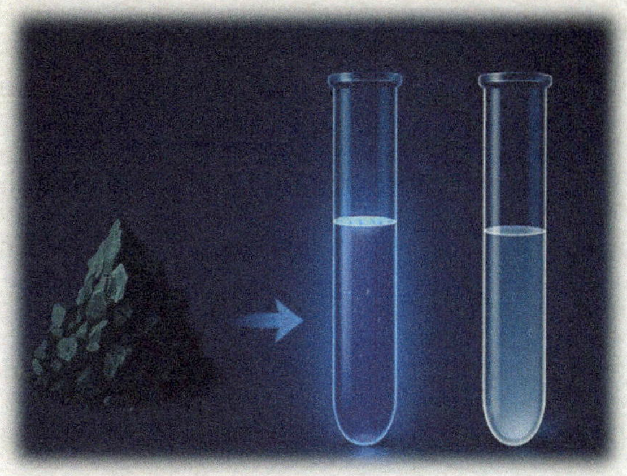

Enhancing mitochondrial function in neurons helps maintain the high energy demands of brain cells. Additionally, methylene blue facilitates the clearance of tau proteins, abnormal accumulations of which are associated with various neurodegenerative conditions[27].

The compound's interaction with cellular metabolism extends to both glucose and fat utilization. By supporting mitochondrial function, methylene blue helps optimize how cells utilize these energy sources[20]. This can lead to improved metabolic efficiency throughout the body, potentially benefiting not only cognitive function but also physical energy levels.

At the molecular level, methylene blue's interaction with the electron transport chain creates a fascinating cascade effect. As it cycles between its oxidized and reduced forms, it helps maintain proper electron flow through the mitochondrial system[20]. This cycling not only supports energy production but also helps prevent the formation of damaging free radicals, effectively acting as an upstream antioxidant[20].

The compound's interaction with cellular systems also includes important effects on inflammation and immune function. Through its modulation of nitric oxide production and other inflammatory mediators[21 22], methylene blue can help regulate immune responses. This property, combined with its direct antimicrobial effects[21], makes it a valuable tool in managing various infectious and inflammatory conditions.

Understanding these biological interactions is crucial for proper therapeutic application. The compound's effects are dose-dependent, with different concentrations producing varying biological responses[26]. At low doses, methylene blue primarily enhances mitochondrial function and provides antioxidant benefits[20]. At higher doses, its effects on enzyme systems and vascular function become more prominent[21 22 26], requiring careful consideration of timing and potential interactions with other medications[23 25].

These diverse biological interactions explain why methylene blue has such wide-ranging therapeutic potential. From supporting cellular energy production to protecting against oxidative stress, and from modulating vascular function to enhancing cognitive performance, the compound's effects stem from its fundamental ability to interact with and optimize crucial biological processes[20] [21] [22]. This understanding continues to drive research into new therapeutic applications while helping to refine existing protocols for maximum safety and efficacy.

Safety Profile and Historical Documentation

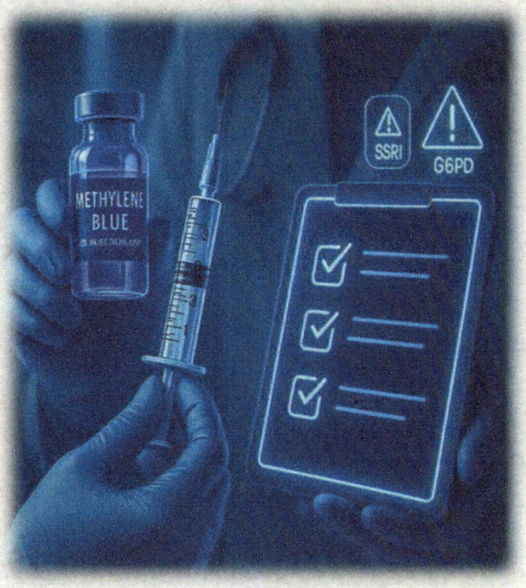

The safety profile of methylene blue spans over a century of documented medical use, providing a wealth of evidence regarding its therapeutic benefits and potential risks. This extensive history, combined with modern research and clinical experience, has established clear guidelines for the safe and effective use of this treatment. Understanding these safety parameters is crucial for anyone considering methylene blue as a therapeutic option.

Methylene blue's safety profile is notably dose-dependent, with different concentrations producing varying biological effects and potential risks[28] [30]. At therapeutic doses, typically ranging from 1 to 2 mg/kg for acute conditions such as methemoglobinemia, the compound demonstrates an excellent safety record when administered properly. However, higher doses can lead to paradoxical effects and increased risk of adverse reactions.

The FDA has approved methylene blue specifically for treating methemoglobinemia, though its use extends to various off-label applications under medical supervision[18]. This regulatory status reflects both its established therapeutic value and the importance of proper medical oversight in its administration. The compound's long history in medical practice has helped establish clear protocols for its safe use, including proper dosing guidelines and important contraindications.

One of the most significant safety considerations involves the interaction of methylene blue with serotonergic medications. As a potent monoamine oxidase inhibitor (MAOI), methylene blue can trigger serotonin syndrome when combined with drugs that affect serotonin levels, such as selective serotonin reuptake inhibitors (SSRIs)[28 18 29 30]. This potentially life-threatening condition requires careful screening of patients' medication histories before administration.

Another crucial safety consideration involves patients with glucose-6-phosphate dehydrogenase (G6PD) deficiency. In these individuals, methylene blue can trigger severe hemolysis, the destruction of red blood cells[30]. This genetic condition affects millions worldwide, making screening for G6PD deficiency an essential step before initiating methylene blue therapy.

Common side effects of methylene blue are generally mild and transient, including temporary discoloration of urine and stool, mild nausea, and dizziness[30]. More serious adverse effects are rare when the compound is administered correctly at therapeutic doses. However, the potential for skin necrosis and local tissue damage at injection sites necessitates proper dilution and careful administration techniques[28].

The historical documentation of methylene blue's safety profile has evolved significantly since its first medical applications in the 1890s. Early research by Paul Ehrlich established its potential as both a diagnostic tool and therapeutic agent, leading to expanded medical applications throughout the 20th century[28]. Modern documentation emphasizes the importance of proper patient screening, adherence to dosing protocols, and close monitoring for potential adverse effects.

Regulatory agencies worldwide have issued specific guidelines regarding methylene blue's use, particularly concerning its interaction with psychiatric medications[23] [29]. These guidelines emphasize the importance of thorough patient assessment and the necessity of proper medical supervision during administration. The compound's interference with pulse oximetry readings also requires special consideration during medical procedures[30].

Long-term safety data from clinical use have helped establish optimal dosing ranges for various applications. Low-dose protocols, typically used for cognitive enhancement and mitochondrial support, have demonstrated particularly favorable safety profiles when properly implemented. However, even at lower doses, adherence to quality standards and proper administration protocols remains essential.

The documentation of methylene blue's safety profile continues to evolve as new research uncovers additional applications and potential interactions[28 18 30]. Current safety protocols emphasize the importance of using pharmaceutical-grade products, maintaining proper storage conditions, and exercising caution when considering contraindications. This growing body of knowledge helps ensure that methylene blue can be used effectively while minimizing potential risks.

Modern safety protocols for methylene blue administration include careful screening for contraindications, proper dose calculation based on body weight and intended use, and monitoring for potential adverse effects[18 30]. Healthcare providers must stay current with the latest guidelines and regulatory updates to ensure optimal patient safety in clinical practice. The compound's extensive safety documentation provides a solid foundation for its continued use in both traditional and emerging therapeutic applications.

Key Historical Milestones in Methylene Blue Research

The scientific journey of methylene blue represents one of medicine's most remarkable examples of how systematic research can transform a simple compound into a powerful therapeutic tool. First synthesized by Heinrich Caro at BASF in 1876[14 1 15 32 16 33], methylene blue began its journey as an industrial textile dye before emerging as a cornerstone of modern medicine. This transition from industrial compound to therapeutic agent would set the stage for numerous groundbreaking discoveries in medical science.

The compound's entry into medical research began in 1880 when microbiologist Robert Koch demonstrated its value as a biological stain for visualizing bacteria under the microscope[15]. This application revolutionized the field of microbiology, providing researchers with an essential tool for studying pathogenic organisms. Koch's work laid the foundation for the broader applications of methylene blue in medical research and diagnostics.

A pivotal moment in methylene blue's history occurred in 1891, when Paul Ehrlich and Paul Guttmann demonstrated its effectiveness against malaria, establishing it as the first fully synthetic drug used in medicine[1 32 16]. This breakthrough marked the birth of modern chemotherapy and the development of synthetic drugs. The success of methylene blue in treating malaria inspired the development of numerous other synthetic drugs, including modern antimalarial like chloroquine[1].

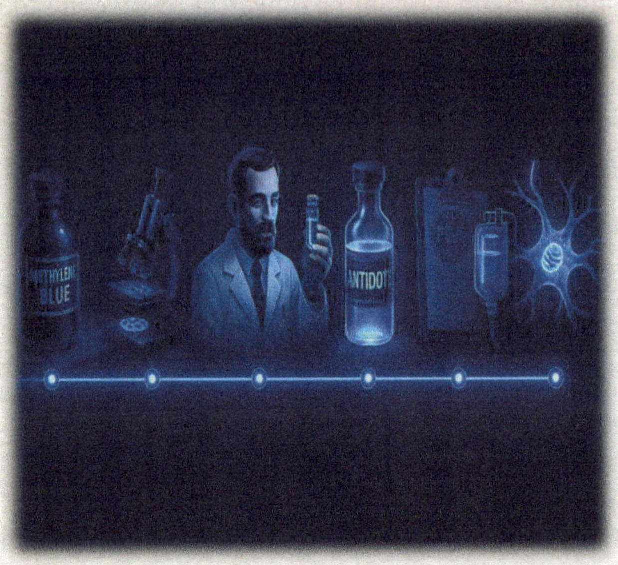

The early 20th century saw rapid expansion in methylene blue research and applications. Its ability to selectively stain tissues and interact with biological systems led to numerous medical innovations. Surgeons began utilizing it for lymph node mapping and tissue visualization during procedures[14 31], while researchers explored its potential in treating various conditions. In 1933, scientist Matilda Brooks made another significant breakthrough, discovering the effectiveness of methylene blue as an antidote for carbon monoxide and cyanide poisoning[1].

The compound's versatility became increasingly apparent as research progressed. Its approval by the FDA in 1950 for treating methemoglobinemia solidified its place in modern medicine[1 32]. This recognition followed extensive documentation of its safety and efficacy in converting abnormal hemoglobin back to its functional form, thereby demonstrating methylene blue's crucial role in emergency medicine.

The latter half of the 20th century brought renewed interest in methylene blue's therapeutic potential. Researchers began investigating its effects on cellular energy production and mitochondrial function, uncovering mechanisms that would explain many of its beneficial effects. These discoveries opened new avenues for research into neurodegenerative conditions, psychiatric disorders, and cellular energy metabolism.

Modern research continues to uncover new applications for methylene blue. Its broad-spectrum antimicrobial properties have gained attention in an era of increasing antibiotic resistance[14 31]. Recent studies have explored its potential antiviral effects, including possible applications against respiratory viruses[31]. Additionally, researchers like Claude Wischik have investigated its potential role in treating neurodegenerative conditions such as Alzheimer's disease[16].

The influence of methylene blue extends beyond its direct applications. As a prototype molecule, it has inspired the development of entire classes of medications, particularly in the fields of antimalarial and antipsychotic drugs[1]. Its unique molecular structure and biological activities continue to serve as a model for drug development and therapeutic innovation.

Contemporary research focuses on optimizing the therapeutic potential of methylene blue while maintaining its remarkable safety profile. Scientists are exploring new delivery methods, investigating potential synergies with other treatments, and developing protocols for various medical applications. This ongoing research continues to reveal new aspects of this versatile compound's therapeutic potential.

The historical milestones in methylene blue research demonstrate the compound's remarkable journey from an industrial dye to a therapeutic agent[16 14 1 32]. Each discovery has contributed to our understanding of its mechanisms and applications, while also inspiring new directions in medical research. As investigations continue, the role of methylene blue in medicine continues to evolve, promising new therapeutic possibilities for future generations.

The Science behind Methylene Blue's Versatility

The remarkable versatility of methylene blue stems from its unique molecular structure and biochemical properties, which enable it to perform multiple functions within biological systems. At its core, methylene blue ($C_{16}H_{18}ClN_3S$) is a small, heterocyclic aromatic compound that can easily cross cell membranes and interact with various cellular components[34 7]. This molecular design enables it to serve as both an electron carrier and a powerful therapeutic agent in various medical applications.

The foundation of methylene blue's versatility lies in its exceptional redox cycling capabilities. In its oxidized form, it appears blue, while its reduced form (leucomethylene blue) is colorless[1 34]. This property isn't merely cosmetic, it represents the compound's ability to accept and donate electrons efficiently within cellular systems. With a redox midpoint potential of +0.01 V1 34, methylene blue can participate in crucial electron transfer processes that support cellular energy production and protect against oxidative stress.

One of methylene blue's most significant features is its ability to serve as an alternative electron carrier in the mitochondrial electron transport chain. When cellular energy production becomes compromised, methylene blue can accept electrons from compounds like NADH and $FADH_2$, then transfer them to cytochrome c. This bypass mechanism helps maintain ATP production while reducing the formation of harmful reactive oxygen species, thereby effectively supporting cellular energy generation and providing antioxidant protection1.

The compound's high water solubility (43,600 mg/L at 25°C) combined with its ability to cross biological barriers, makes it exceptionally effective in various therapeutic applications[34 12]. Its molecular weight of 319.85 g/mol enables it to readily cross the blood-brain barrier, allowing for direct interaction with neural tissues. This property, coupled with its ability to carry electrons, explains its potential in treating various neurological conditions and supporting cognitive function.

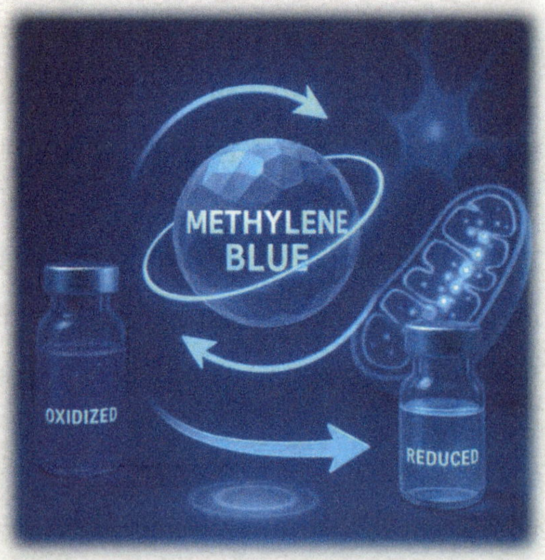

Methylene blue's interaction with biological systems extends beyond its role as an electron carrier. The compound can inhibit certain enzymes, including soluble guanylyl cyclase, and prevent tau protein aggregation—processes implicated in various pathological conditions. These mechanisms contribute to its potential therapeutic applications in neurodegenerative disorders and cardiovascular health[7].

The compound's spectral properties, particularly its strong absorption near 664-670 nm, enable its use in both diagnostic and therapeutic applications[134]. This characteristic absorption pattern allows methylene blue to function effectively in photodynamic therapy and various analytical procedures. When exposed to specific wavelengths of light, it can produce reactive oxygen species, making it valuable in antimicrobial and cancer treatments[7].

Understanding the chemical versatility of methylene blue helps explain its broad range of therapeutic applications. Its ability to participate in redox reactions while maintaining stability under normal conditions makes it a reliable tool in medical practice. However, this same versatility requires careful attention to proper dosing and administration, as its effects can vary significantly depending on the concentration and application method[8 7].

The compound's aggregation behavior at higher concentrations, forming dimers and trimers, influences its therapeutic effectiveness[1]. This property necessitates careful consideration of dosing protocols to achieve optimal results. Additionally, its interaction with cellular components can be concentration-dependent, with different doses producing varying biological responses.

Methylene blue's versatility in medical applications continues to expand as research uncovers new therapeutic potential. From its traditional use in treating methemoglobinemia to emerging applications in neurodegenerative disorders, the compound's fundamental properties enable a wide range of therapeutic interventions[34]. However, this versatility must be balanced with careful attention to safety considerations and potential interactions with other medications[8 7].

The scientific understanding of methylene blue's versatility provides a solid foundation for its therapeutic applications while highlighting the importance of proper protocols and safety measures. As research continues to reveal new applications, the compound's fundamental properties—its redox activity, membrane permeability, and enzyme interactions—remain central to its therapeutic potential[17]. This understanding enables healthcare practitioners to leverage methylene blue's versatility effectively while maintaining appropriate safety standards and optimizing therapeutic outcomes.

As we conclude this initial chapter exploring the science and history of methylene blue, we've uncovered the remarkable journey of a compound that has profoundly impacted modern medicine. From its serendipitous discovery as a textile dye to its evolution into a versatile therapeutic agent, methylene blue continues to demonstrate its value in countless medical applications. Its unique molecular structure and ability to enhance cellular energy production make it a fascinating subject for ongoing research and practical applications.

Through our exploration, we've discovered how methylene blue's fundamental properties, its electron-carrying capabilities, ability to cross biological barriers, and interaction with cellular processes create the foundation for its diverse therapeutic potential. We've traced its historical development from the first synthetic drug used in medicine to its current status as a valuable tool in emergency medicine, surgical procedures, and emerging therapeutic protocols.

By understanding the basic chemistry and biological interactions of methylene blue, we've gained crucial insights into how this remarkable compound supports cellular health and energy production. Its ability to enhance mitochondrial function while providing antioxidant protection demonstrates why it continues to attract attention in both traditional medical applications and cutting-edge research.

Key insights from this chapter include:

- Methylene blue's unique molecular structure enables it to function as both an electron carrier and a therapeutic agent

- The compound's ability to cross the blood-brain barrier makes it valuable for neurological applications

- Its historical development has led to numerous medical breakthroughs and inspired modern drug development

- A proper understanding of its mechanisms and safety profile is essential for therapeutic success

- The compound's versatility stems from its fundamental chemical properties and biological interactions

Moving into methylene blue's specific benefits and applications, this foundational understanding provides the framework for effectively harnessing its therapeutic potential. The transformation from industrial dye to medical breakthrough highlights the value of continuous scientific inquiry and precise protocol development in maximizing its benefits while maintaining safety.

Remember that while methylene blue shows remarkable promise across various applications, its use requires proper knowledge of dosing, safety considerations, and potential interactions. This understanding forms the basis for the responsible and effective implementation of methylene blue therapy, whether in clinical settings or personal health protocols.

In the chapters ahead, we'll delve deeper into specific applications and benefits of methylene blue, building upon this fundamental knowledge to explore practical protocols and therapeutic strategies. The groundwork laid in this chapter will serve as a crucial reference point as we examine how this versatile compound can be effectively utilized to support health and healing across various conditions and applications.

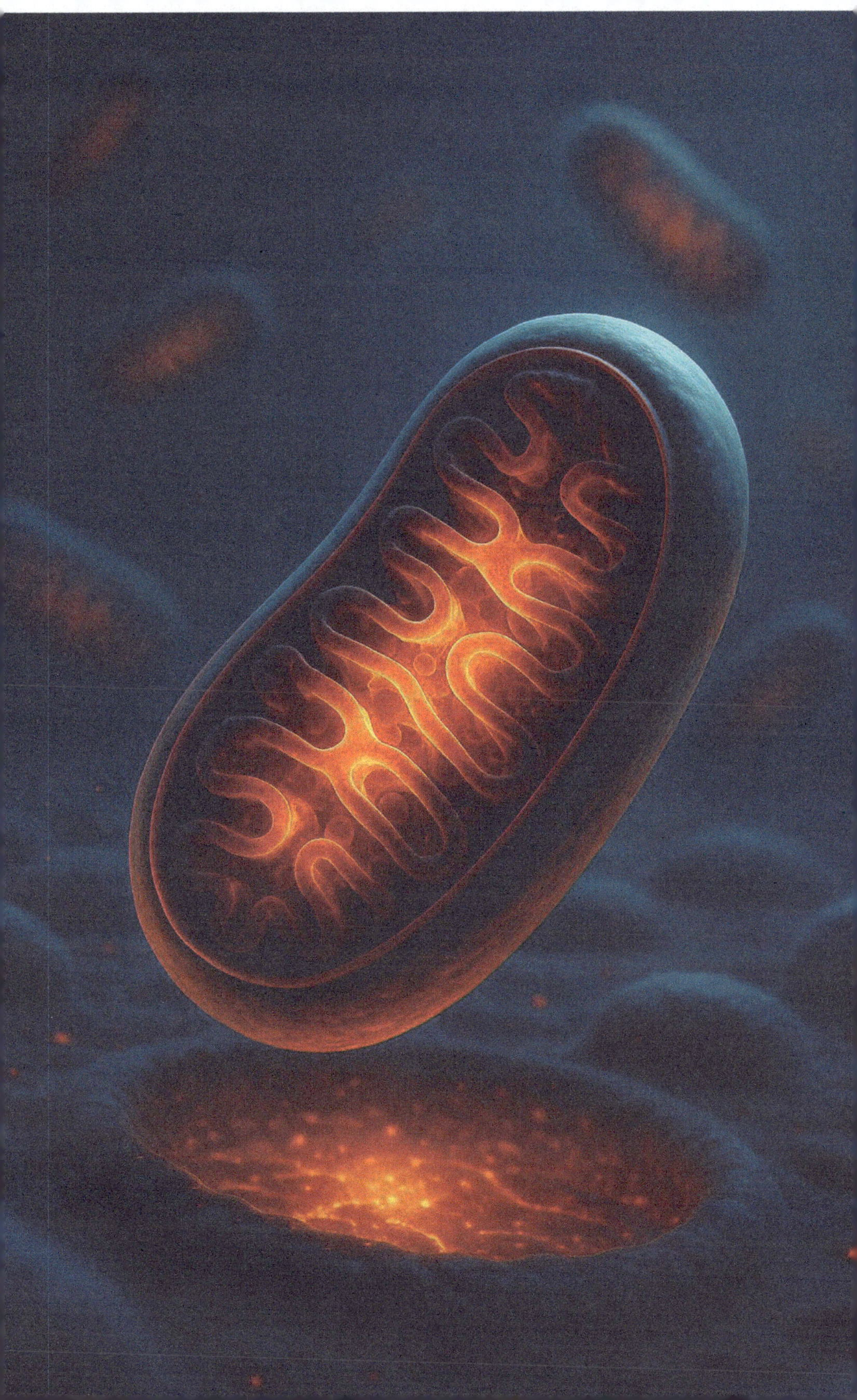

CHAPTER 2

THE CELLULAR POWER PLANT: HOW METHYLENE BLUE ENERGIZES YOUR MITOCHONDRIA

Deep within each of your cells lies an intricate network of microscopic power plants, the mitochondria, tirelessly working to keep you energized and alive. These remarkable organelles hold the key to understanding one of methylene blue's most profound benefits: its ability to enhance cellular energy production in ways that conventional supplements simply cannot match. Methylene blue's extraordinary effect on mitochondria represents one of its most significant therapeutic applications, positioning it as a unique and powerful tool for cellular rejuvenation. At the heart of this mechanism lies its ability to serve as an alternative electron carrier in the electron transport chain, effectively bypassing damaged or inefficient pathways to optimize energy production.

Understanding how methylene blue interacts with mitochondria reveals why this molecule stands apart from conventional supplements and medications. Unlike standard antioxidants that neutralize free radicals, methylene blue actively participates in cellular energy production. It acts as a molecular "shuttle," efficiently transferring electrons within the mitochondria's intricate machinery.

The implications of this cellular enhancement extend far beyond simple energy production. When mitochondrial function improves, every system in the body benefits - from cognitive performance to physical endurance. This chapter will examine the intricate relationship between methylene blue and cellular energy production, breaking down complex biochemical processes into practical and applicable knowledge.

In the following sections, we'll examine how methylene blue optimizes mitochondrial function, increases ATP production, and supports overall cellular health. We'll also discuss practical applications for addressing fatigue, enhancing physical performance, and supporting healthy aging through improved mitochondrial function. Understanding these mechanisms is crucial for anyone looking to harness the full potential of methylene blue for health optimization.

Most importantly, we'll explore how this remarkable molecule can be used effectively and safely to support mitochondrial health, with a specific focus on dosing strategies and potential contraindications. This knowledge will empower you to make informed decisions about incorporating methylene blue into your health protocol, understanding not only what it does but also how to optimize its benefits for your specific needs.

Understanding Mitochondria: Your Cellular Energy Factories

To truly understand how methylene blue enhances cellular function, we must first explore the remarkable world of mitochondria, the microscopic powerhouses that fuel every cell in the body[35 38 41]. These tiny but mighty organelles are responsible for producing about 90% of the energy your cells need to function, making them central to health, vitality, and longevity.

Mitochondria are unique among cellular structures because they have their own DNA and two distinct membranes: an outer membrane and an intricately folded inner membrane[38]. This double-membrane structure is crucial for energy production through a process known as oxidative phosphorylation[37]. The inner membrane contains the electron transport chain, a series of protein complexes that work together like a molecular assembly line to produce adenosine triphosphate (ATP), the primary energy currency of cells[37 42].

The number of mitochondria in each cell varies depending on that cell's energy requirements. Cells with high energy demands, such as those in the brain, muscles, liver, and kidneys, can contain thousands of mitochondria, while other cells may have only a few hundred[35 38]. This variable distribution highlights why certain tissues are particularly responsive to compounds that enhance mitochondrial function, like methylene blue.

Mitochondria generate energy through a complex process known as cellular respiration. This multi-step pathway breaks down nutrients from the food we eat—primarily glucose, fatty acids, and amino acids into a usable form of energy (ATP)[35 36 37 39 40 42]. Without mitochondria, cells would be forced to rely on less efficient energy-producing processes, generating only a fraction of the ATP needed for optimal function[37 42].

The electron transport chain within mitochondria is particularly noteworthy because it's where methylene blue exerts many of its beneficial effects. This chain consists of five protein complexes that pass electrons from one to another, much like a molecular game of hot potato. As electrons move through this chain, they generate a proton gradient that drives ATP production[37]. When this process becomes inefficient due to age, disease, or environmental factors, cellular energy production suffers.

Beyond energy production, mitochondria serve as central hubs for numerous other vital cellular processes. They help regulate cell death (apoptosis), manage reactive oxygen species, and facilitate the metabolism of various nutrients[36 39]. The health of your mitochondria is inextricably linked to aging, cognitive function, physical performance, and overall well-being[35 39].

Understanding mitochondrial function is crucial because dysfunction in these organelles is associated with a wide range of health conditions.

From neurodegenerative diseases to metabolic disorders, compromised mitochondrial function can have far-reaching effects on health[38 43]. This is where methylene blue's ability to optimize mitochondrial function becomes particularly relevant.

Mitochondria also play a crucial role in managing cellular stress by regulating the handling of reactive oxygen species (ROS). While ROS are natural byproducts of energy production, excessive amounts can damage cellular components[39]. Healthy mitochondria maintain a delicate balance between energy production and ROS management, a balance that methylene blue helps optimize.

The efficiency of mitochondrial function naturally declines with age, contributing to various age-related health challenges[35 39]. This decline affects everything from energy levels and cognitive function to physical performance and cellular repair processes. Supporting mitochondrial health through interventions like methylene blue represents a promising strategy for maintaining vitality as we age.

Perhaps most remarkably, mitochondria can adapt their function in response to cellular demands and environmental conditions. This adaptability, known as mitochondrial plasticity, enables cells to respond to fluctuating energy demands and stress levels. Understanding this dynamic nature helps explain why compounds that support mitochondrial function can have such profound effects on overall health and performance.

The Electron Transport Chain: Where Methylene Blue Works Its Magic

The electron transport chain (ETC) represents one of the most fascinating intersections between methylene blue and cellular energy production. This intricate system, embedded within the inner mitochondrial membrane, serves as the primary site where methylene blue performs its remarkable energy-enhancing effects[44 45 46]. Think of the ETC as a molecular assembly line, where electrons are passed from one complex to another in a carefully orchestrated dance that ultimately powers your cells.

At its core, the electron transport chain consists of five protein complexes (I through V) that work together to generate cellular energy in the form of ATP. Under normal conditions, electrons flow through these complexes like a molecular game of hot potato, with each transfer driving the pumping of protons across the membrane. This proton gradient ultimately powers ATP synthesis, much like water flowing over a dam generates electricity[44].

Methylene blue's unique interaction with the electron transport chain sets it apart from other supplements and therapeutic compounds. Its ability to cycle between oxidized and reduced states allows it to serve as both an electron donor and acceptor—a property known as redox cycling[44 45 46]. This distinctive characteristic enables methylene blue to act as a molecular shuttle, bypassing potential blockages or inefficiencies in the normal electron transport pathway.

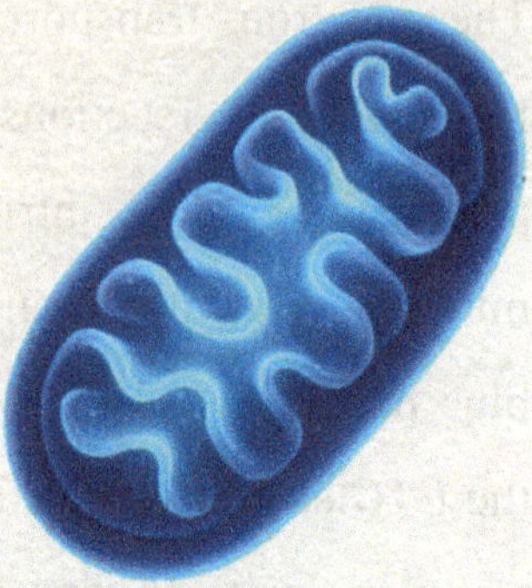

One of methylene blue's most remarkable features is its ability to accept electrons from NADH and $FADH_2$, then deliver them directly to cytochrome c, effectively creating an alternative pathway when the conventional route is compromised[46 47 48]. This bypass mechanism becomes particularly valuable in situations where the normal electron transport chain function is impaired, such as in aging, neurodegenerative conditions, or cellular stress[45 46].

The implications of this alternative electron transport pathway are profound. By maintaining electron flow even when conventional pathways are compromised, methylene blue helps sustain ATP production while simultaneously reducing the formation of harmful reactive oxygen species (ROS)[45 46]. This dual action of energy support and protection makes it a powerful tool for optimizing cellular health.

Low-dose methylene blue has been shown to stimulate mitochondrial oxygen consumption and enhance the activity of cytochrome oxidase

(Complex IV), resulting in increased ATP synthesis[44]. Perhaps even more importantly, it can upregulate the expression of cytochrome oxidase subunits, promoting long-term improvements in mitochondrial energy metabolism and cellular resilience[44].

The efficiency of methylene blue's interaction with the electron transport chain has been demonstrated in numerous scientific studies. Research has shown that it can effectively bypass blockages caused by various toxins and metabolic inhibitors, helping to restore electron transport chain function and protect against cellular damage[46]. This protective effect has been observed in models of neurodegenerative disease and mitochondrial injury[44 46].

In the context of brain health, the effects of methylene blue on the electron transport chain become particularly significant. Studies have demonstrated its ability to increase cerebral metabolic rate and oxygen utilization, supporting brain energy metabolism even under challenging conditions such as hypoxia[44]. This makes it a promising compound for supporting cognitive function and neurological health.

The practical implications of methylene blue's effects on the electron transport chain extend beyond basic cellular function. By optimizing energy production at the molecular level, it can influence everything from physical endurance to mental clarity[44 45]. However, it's crucial to note that these benefits are typically observed at low to moderate doses, as higher concentrations may actually inhibit electron transport chain function.

Understanding the role of methylene blue in the electron transport chain helps explain its broad spectrum of potential therapeutic applications. From supporting healthy aging to enhancing cognitive function, its ability to optimize cellular energy production through the electron transport chain makes it a unique and valuable tool in the pursuit of optimal health and vitality.

ATP Production: Boosting Your Cellular Energy Currency

At the heart of cellular energy production lies ATP (adenosine triphosphate), the molecular currency that powers virtually every biological process in your body. This remarkable molecule serves as the universal energy carrier, fueling everything from muscle contractions to nerve signaling, and from cellular repair to the synthesis of vital compounds[50]. Understanding how methylene blue enhances ATP production reveals why this compound has such profound effects on cellular vitality and overall health.

The relationship between methylene blue and ATP production is particularly fascinating because it operates through multiple complementary mechanisms. When methylene blue enters the cell, it can significantly enhance ATP production by up to 30% through its unique ability to improve electron transport chain efficiency[20]. This improvement in energy output isn't just a temporary boost, it represents a fundamental optimization of cellular energy metabolism.

Methylene blue's ability to enhance ATP production stems from its role as an alternative electron carrier in the mitochondrial electron transport chain. By accepting electrons from NADH and $FADH_2$ and delivering them directly to cytochrome c, methylene blue creates an efficient bypass around potential blockages or inefficiencies in the normal electron transport pathway[20 49 50]. This process is particularly valuable when conventional pathways are compromised due to age, disease, or environmental stressors[49].

The implications of enhanced ATP production extend far beyond simple energy availability. When cells have access to abundant ATP, they can maintain optimal function across all systems - from cellular repair and protein synthesis to neurotransmitter production and membrane maintenance. This increased energy availability is particularly crucial for high-energy cells, such as the brain, heart, and muscles[20 50.]

Methylene blue's impact on ATP production becomes even more significant under conditions of cellular stress or metabolic challenge. Research has demonstrated that low doses of methylene blue can increase cellular oxygen consumption by up to 70%, resulting in enhanced ATP synthesis[20]. This improvement in energy production efficiency helps cells maintain vital functions even under challenging conditions.

One of the most remarkable aspects of methylene blue's effect on ATP production is its ability to support sustained energy output while simultaneously reducing oxidative stress. Unlike many interventions that boost energy at the cost of increased free radical production, methylene blue's unique redox cycling properties allow it to enhance ATP synthesis while actually decreasing oxidative damage[20 51]. This dual action makes it particularly valuable for long-term cellular health optimization.

The practical implications of enhanced ATP production through methylene blue supplementation are far-reaching. From supporting cognitive function and mental clarity to enhancing physical performance and recovery, optimal ATP levels are fundamental to health and vitality[49]. However, it's crucial to note that these benefits are typically observed at low to moderate doses, as higher concentrations may actually inhibit electron transport chain function.

For cells with high energy demands, such as neurons, the ATP-enhancing effects of methylene blue can be particularly beneficial. By ensuring a steady supply of cellular energy, methylene blue helps support critical processes such as neurotransmission, synaptic plasticity, and cellular repair[20 50]. This enhanced energy availability may help explain many of methylene blue's documented cognitive and neuroprotective benefits.

The optimization of ATP production through methylene blue supplementation represents a fundamental approach to supporting cellular health and function. Rather than simply providing temporary stimulation or masking fatigue, methylene blue works at the molecular level to enhance the body's natural energy-producing capabilities[49]. This enhancement of cellular energetics can contribute to improved resilience, better stress tolerance, and more efficient cellular repair processes.

When implementing methylene blue for ATP enhancement, it's essential to consider proper dosing and timing. Research indicates that low doses (0.5-4 mg/kg) are most effective for optimizing ATP production without risking inhibitory effects[20 50]. Additionally, the timing of administration can be coordinated with periods of high energy demand to maximize benefits while maintaining safety and effectiveness.

Oxidative Stress and Mitochondrial Protection

The intricate balance between oxidative stress and cellular health represents one of the most critical battlegrounds in the pursuit of optimal wellness and longevity. Within our cells, particularly in the mitochondria, a constant struggle unfolds between the production of harmful free radicals and our body's natural antioxidant defenses[20]. Methylene blue emerges as a powerful ally in this molecular warfare, offering unique protective properties that set it apart from conventional antioxidants.

Oxidative stress occurs when our bodies produce more reactive oxygen species (ROS) than they can effectively neutralize. This imbalance leads to cellular damage and contributes to numerous health conditions, including neurodegenerative diseases, cardiovascular problems, and accelerated aging[52]. The mitochondria, while essential for energy production, are particularly vulnerable to oxidative damage due to their role in electron transport and ATP synthesis[20].

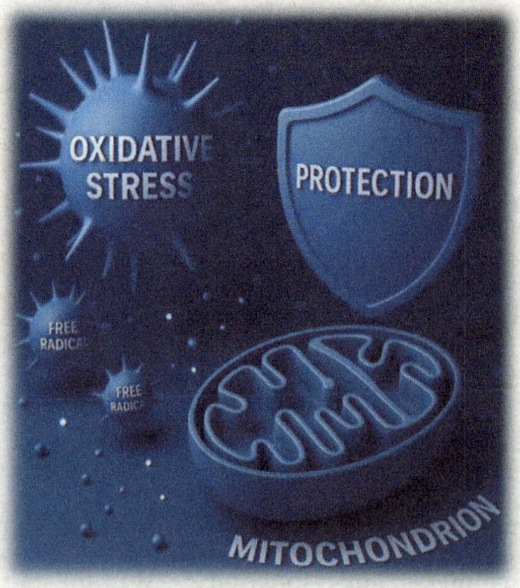

Methylene blue's protective capabilities extend far beyond simple antioxidant activity. Its unique molecular structure allows it to act as a renewable electron shuttle, effectively preventing the formation of harmful ROS at their source rather than merely neutralizing them after they've formed[20 52]. This proactive approach to oxidative stress management represents a significant advancement in cellular protection strategies.

One of methylene blue's most remarkable features is its ability to enhance mitochondrial function while simultaneously reducing oxidative stress[52 53]. Supporting smooth electron flow through the electron transport chain, it helps prevent the electron leakage that typically leads to ROS formation[20]. This dual action of optimization and protection makes it particularly valuable for maintaining cellular health.

The implications of methylene blue's protective effects are particularly significant for high-energy organs, such as the brain, heart, and muscles. These tissues, with their abundant mitochondria and high energy demands, are especially susceptible to oxidative damage. Methylene blue's ability to cross the blood-brain barrier makes it particularly effective in supporting neurological health and cognitive function[53].

Research has demonstrated that methylene blue's antioxidant properties extend beyond direct ROS neutralization. It also helps stabilize mitochondrial function and supports DNA repair mechanisms, providing comprehensive cellular protection[52]. This multifaceted approach to cellular defense helps explain its broad spectrum of potential therapeutic applications.

When implementing methylene blue for oxidative stress protection, dosing considerations become crucial. Low doses have been shown to provide optimal benefits, while higher doses may actually increase oxidative stress. This hormetic effect highlights the importance of adhering to proper dosing protocols and seeking professional guidance when using methylene blue therapeutically.

The protective benefits of methylene blue are particularly relevant in the context of aging and age-related diseases. As we age, our natural antioxidant defenses typically decline, making supplemental support increasingly important. Methylene blue's ability to support mitochondrial function while reducing oxidative stress makes it a promising tool for healthy aging strategies[53 54].

Perhaps most significantly, methylene blue's protective effects appear to be self-renewing due to its ability to cycle between oxidized and reduced states[20 52]. This unique characteristic allows it to provide sustained protection against oxidative stress, unlike conventional antioxidants that become depleted after neutralizing free radicals. This renewable protection makes it particularly valuable for maintaining long-term cellular health.

Understanding the role of methylene blue in protecting against oxidative stress and promoting mitochondrial health provides crucial insights into its therapeutic potential. From supporting cognitive function to enhancing cellular resilience, its unique mechanisms of action offer promising applications across a wide range of health conditions[53]. However, it's essential to approach its use with careful consideration of proper dosing and individual health factors to maximize its benefits while ensuring safety.

Methylene Blue as an Alternative Electron Carrier

Methylene blue's remarkable ability to serve as an alternative electron carrier distinguishes it from conventional supplements and therapeutic compounds[50 45 46]. This unique property allows it to enhance cellular energy production in ways that other interventions cannot match. By acting as a molecular shuttle within the mitochondria, methylene blue creates an efficient bypass around potential blockages or inefficiencies in the electron transport chain, thereby effectively optimizing cellular energy production[55 46].

At its core, methylene blue functions through a sophisticated process called redox cycling, where it alternates between its oxidized (MB+) and reduced (leucomethylene blue) forms. This cycling enables methylene blue to accept electrons from critical molecules, such as NADH, NADPH, and $FADH_2$, and then deliver them directly to cytochrome c[50 1 46]. This direct delivery system creates an alternative pathway for electron flow, particularly valuable when the conventional electron transport chain is compromised due to age, disease, or environmental stressors[45 46].

The implications of this alternative electron transport mechanism are profound. By maintaining efficient electron flow even when conventional pathways are impaired, methylene blue helps sustain ATP production while simultaneously reducing the formation of harmful reactive oxygen species[55]. This dual action of energy support and protection makes it a powerful tool for optimizing cellular health.

Research has demonstrated that methylene blue's electron carrier capabilities become particularly significant under conditions of cellular stress or metabolic challenge. Its ability to bypass impaired complexes I and III of the electron transport chain while directly reducing cytochrome c represents a crucial metabolic rescue mechanism[55 46]. This property has shown promise in various models of mitochondrial dysfunction, including neurodegenerative conditions and age-related decline[45 46 56].

Perhaps most remarkably, methylene blue's electron carrier function extends beyond simple energy production. By providing an alternative route for electrons, it helps limit electron leakage, which typically leads to oxidative damage[55]. This reduction in oxidative stress, combined with enhanced energy production, creates a synergistic effect that supports overall cellular health and function.

The molecular properties that enable methylene blue to serve as an effective electron carrier are equally fascinating. Its redox midpoint potential of +0.01 V allows for efficient interaction with biological redox systems, while its small size and lipophilicity enable it to cross cellular and mitochondrial membranes easily[45 1]. These characteristics make methylene blue uniquely suited for its role in cellular energy optimization.

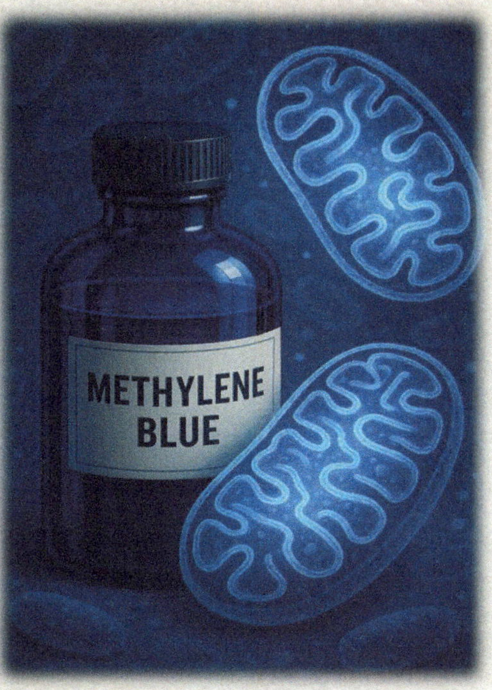

When implementing methylene blue as an alternative electron carrier, proper dosing becomes crucial. Research indicates that low doses are most effective for optimizing electron transport chain function without risking inhibitory effects. This hormetic response highlights the importance of adhering to careful dosing protocols and seeking professional guidance when using methylene blue therapeutically.

The practical applications of methylene blue's electron carrier properties extend across various therapeutic contexts. From supporting cognitive function and neuroprotection to enhancing cellular resilience and metabolic health, its unique mechanism of action offers promising applications for various health conditions[45 56]. However, it's essential to approach its use with careful consideration of proper dosing and individual health factors.

Understanding the role of methylene blue as an alternative electron carrier provides crucial insights into its therapeutic potential. Its ability to optimize cellular energy production while simultaneously reducing oxidative stress represents a significant advancement in cellular health optimization[50 45 46]. This dual mechanism of action, combined with its ability to cross cellular membranes and interact efficiently with biological systems, makes it a valuable tool in the pursuit of optimal health and vitality.

For healthcare practitioners and individuals interested in implementing methylene blue therapy, recognizing its function as an alternative electron carrier is fundamental to understanding its proper application. This knowledge helps inform appropriate dosing strategies, timing of administration, and potential contraindications, ensuring safe and effective use of this remarkable compound.

Dosing Strategies for Optimal Mitochondrial Function

Determining the optimal dose of methylene blue for mitochondrial support requires careful consideration of several key factors. Research has consistently shown that methylene blue exhibits a hormetic dose-response, meaning that while low doses enhance mitochondrial function, higher doses may actually impair cellular energy production[59 60]. This unique characteristic makes proper dosing strategies crucial for achieving optimal therapeutic benefits.

The scientific evidence points to a clear distinction between low-dose and high-dose applications. For mitochondrial support and general health optimization, research indicates that doses between 0.5 and 4 mg/kg body weight are most effective[50]. This typically translates to daily doses of 4-30 mg for most adults[59 60 61]. At these lower doses, methylene blue effectively enhances electron transport chain function while minimizing the risk of adverse effects.

Starting with the lowest effective dose is crucial when implementing methylene blue supplementation. A conservative approach begins with 4-8 mg daily, allowing for careful observation of the individual's response before any dose adjustments[57 59 61]. This "start low, go slow" methodology helps establish optimal personal dosing while minimizing the risk of adverse effects.

The timing of administration can significantly impact the effectiveness of methylene blue in supporting mitochondria. Morning dosing often proves most beneficial, as it aligns with natural circadian rhythms and energy demands. However, some individuals may benefit from strategic timing around specific activities or periods of high cognitive demand.

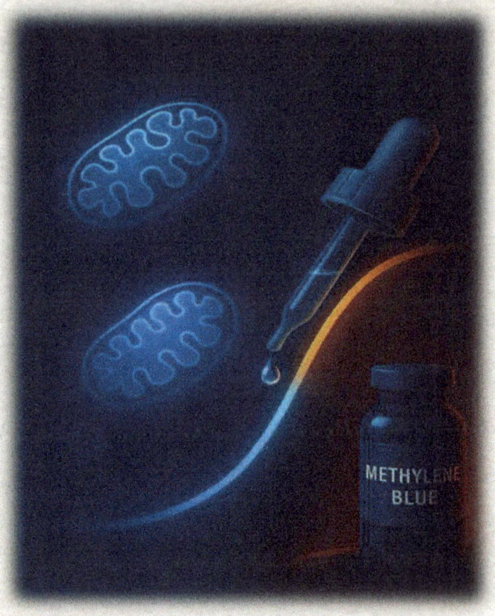

The concentration of the methylene blue solution is another critical consideration. Pharmaceutical-grade methylene blue is typically available in a 1% solution (10 mg/mL), although other concentrations are also available. Accurate measurement becomes essential, as even small variations can significantly impact effectiveness. Using precise measuring tools, such as calibrated droppers or oral syringes, helps ensure consistent dosing.

It's crucial to understand that higher doses (above 100 mg) are reserved for specific medical emergencies in hospital settings and are not appropriate for general mitochondrial support[60]. These higher doses can actually inhibit mitochondrial function and increase oxidative stress, underscoring the importance of staying within the therapeutic window for optimal mitochondrial function.

Safety considerations must remain paramount when implementing methylene blue supplementation. Certain individuals should exercise particular caution or avoid use entirely, including those with G6PD deficiency, pregnancy, or those taking serotonergic medications[57 60]. The risk of serotonin syndrome becomes significant with higher doses or when combined with certain medications.

Dose adjustments may be necessary based on individual factors such as body weight, overall health status, and specific therapeutic goals[57]. Regular monitoring and assessment of response help optimize the dosing strategy over time. Some individuals may achieve optimal results with intermittent dosing rather than daily administration.

The quality and purity of methylene blue significantly impact its effectiveness and safety profile. Pharmaceutical-grade methylene blue (USP grade) ensures the absence of harmful contaminants and consistent potency. Lower-quality sources may contain toxic impurities or inconsistent concentrations, which can compromise both safety and efficacy.

For cognitive enhancement and neuroprotection, research suggests that maintaining consistent low-dose supplementation may be more beneficial than sporadic high-dose administration[59 60 62]. This approach supports steady optimization of mitochondrial function while minimizing potential side effects or adaptation responses.

Practical implementation requires attention to the proper storage and handling of methylene blue solutions. Protection from light and heat helps maintain potency, while proper dilution techniques ensure accurate dosing. Documentation of dosing schedules and responses can help optimize individual protocols over time.

Dosing Protocol Summary:

- Initial dose: 4-8 mg daily[57 59 61]
- Therapeutic range: 4-30 mg daily[59 60 61]
- Optimal timing: Morning administration
- Frequency: Daily or as directed by healthcare provider
- Duration: Ongoing with periodic assessment
- Contraindications: G6PD deficiency, pregnancy, serotonergic medications[57 60]

By following these evidence-based dosing strategies while maintaining awareness of individual factors and safety considerations, methylene blue can be effectively utilized to support optimal mitochondrial function and cellular health[58 61 51]. Regular monitoring and adjustment of protocols ensures maximum benefit while minimizing potential risks.

Age-Related Mitochondrial Decline and Methylene Blue

As we age, our cells face a progressive decline in their ability to generate energy efficiently, largely due to deteriorating mitochondrial function. This fundamental aspect of aging affects every tissue in the body, but has a particularly significant impact on organs with high energy demands, such as the brain, heart, and muscles. Understanding how methylene blue can help combat this decline reveals one of its most promising therapeutic applications for healthy aging.

Mitochondrial dysfunction represents a unifying pathological phenomenon across numerous age-related conditions and neurodegenerative disorders[63]. As cells age, both the number and efficiency of mitochondria decrease, creating a progressive energy deficit that compromises cellular function across multiple organ systems. This decline creates a destructive cycle in which reduced energy production leads to increased oxidative stress, which in turn further damages mitochondrial function. Research has documented that mitochondrial dysfunction occurs in systemic aging, affecting multiple tissues, including the brain and skin[61].

The brain proves especially vulnerable to this age-related mitochondrial decline. Despite comprising only 2% of body weight, the brain consumes approximately 20% of the body's oxygen and glucose. When mitochondrial output drops, neurons struggle to maintain energy-intensive processes required for neurotransmitter synthesis, synaptic transmission, and ion gradient maintenance. This energy crisis contributes significantly to age-related cognitive decline and increases vulnerability to neurodegenerative conditions.

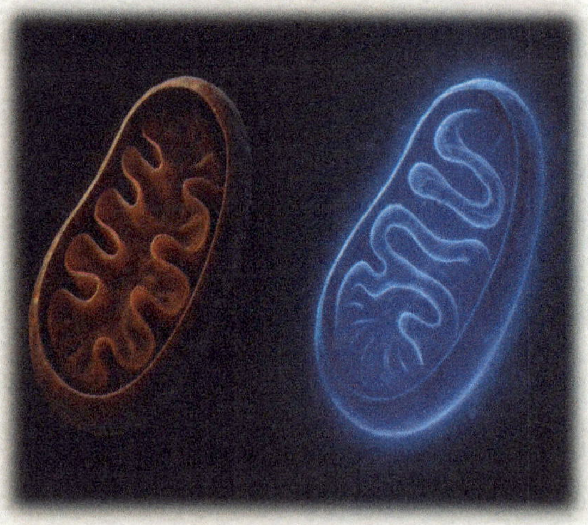

Methylene blue offers a unique solution to this age-related decline through its sophisticated mechanism as an alternative electron carrier within the electron transport chain. It provides a bypass route when normal mitochondrial complexes become damaged or inefficient due to aging. Research has shown that low doses of methylene blue can increase cellular oxygen consumption by up to 70% and boost ATP production by approximately 30%, even in aged or damaged cells[20].

Specifically, methylene blue can reroute electrons in the mitochondrial electron transport chain directly from NADH to cytochrome c, thereby increasing the activity of complex IV and effectively promoting mitochondrial activity while mitigating oxidative stress[63 61]. This bypass mechanism proves crucial because it enables cells to maintain ATP production even when upstream complexes in the electron transport chain have become compromised due to age-related damage.

The compound's unique ability to cycle between its oxidized blue form and reduced colorless form (leucomethylene blue) enables it to act as a renewable antioxidant rather than a single-use compound[20]. This continuous cycling helps buffer redox imbalances and reduce oxidative stress at its source, addressing two fundamental drivers of cellular aging simultaneously.

In both cell culture and animal models, methylene blue maintains its ability to support cellular respiration even in low-oxygen environments—a common problem in aging tissues due to compromised blood flow. Functional MRI studies demonstrate that methylene blue facilitates the conversion of oxygen to water more efficiently, thereby maintaining neuronal function even under hypoxic stress[20]. This increased oxygen efficiency can trigger additional benefits through the production of nitric oxide, which dilates blood vessels and increases blood flow to metabolically active regions[20].

The implications for age-related cognitive decline are particularly significant. Current findings suggest that methylene blue may provide targeted metabolic support to neurons operating at peak load, potentially enhancing memory consolidation and alleviating harmful metabolic stress[20]. This concept of targeted support has generated interest in methylene blue's potential to focus on "energy hotspots" in the brain—regions with high metabolic demands that prove especially vulnerable to age-related decline.

Practical implementation for addressing age-related mitochondrial decline requires careful attention to dosing and timing. Research indicates that doses between 0.5 and 4 mg/kg body weight are most effective for mitochondrial support20, typically translating to daily doses of 4-30 mg for most adults. Morning administration often proves most beneficial, as it aligns with natural circadian rhythms and energy demands.

Safety considerations remain paramount, particularly given the extended duration of use required for addressing age-related decline. Methylene blue's well-established safety profile, derived from over 120 years of clinical use, provides confidence in its long-term safety that newer compounds cannot match63. However, certain individuals should exercise caution, including those with G6PD deficiency or those taking serotonergic medications.

Protocol Summary for Age-Related Mitochondrial Support:

- Initial dose: 4-8 mg daily
- Therapeutic range: 4-30 mg daily

- Optimal timing: Morning administration
- Duration: Ongoing with periodic assessment
- Quality requirement: Pharmaceutical-grade (USP) methylene blue
- Regular monitoring of response and adjustment as needed
- Contraindications: G6PD deficiency, serotonergic medications

Energy Enhancement: From Cellular to Systemic Benefits

The remarkable journey of methylene blue's energy-enhancing effects begins at the cellular level but extends throughout the entire body, creating a cascade of benefits that can transform overall health and vitality. Understanding this progression from cellular to systemic benefits reveals why methylene blue stands apart as a unique therapeutic compound for energy optimization.

At its foundation, methylene blue's cellular energy enhancement occurs through its sophisticated interaction with mitochondrial function. By serving as an alternative electron carrier in the electron transport chain[49 64 45 20], it increases cellular oxygen consumption by up to 70% and boosts ATP production by approximately 30%[45 20]. This fundamental improvement in cellular energetics lays the groundwork for system-wide benefits.

The enhanced cellular energy production translates into improved organ function, particularly in tissues with high energy demands. The brain, heart, and muscles all rich in mitochondria show marked performance improvements when cellular energy production is optimized[64 20]. This enhancement manifests as improved cognitive function, better physical endurance, and enhanced cardiovascular efficiency.

One of the most significant aspects of methylene blue's systemic benefits is its ability to improve energy production while simultaneously reducing oxidative stress[49 64 45 20]. This dual action creates a positive feedback loop where increased energy availability supports better cellular repair and maintenance, while reduced oxidative damage helps preserve cellular function. The result is a comprehensive enhancement of systemic vitality.

The implications for brain function are particularly noteworthy. Enhanced cellular energy in neurons supports everything from neurotransmitter production to synaptic plasticity[64 20]. This improvement in neural energetics translates into better cognitive performance, enhanced memory formation, and improved mental clarity. The brain's high energy demands make it exceptionally responsive to methylene blue's optimization of cellular energy production.

Physical performance benefits emerge as cellular energy enhancement extends to muscular tissue. Improved ATP availability supports better muscle function, enhanced endurance, and faster recovery from physical exertion[49 64]. This improvement in physical capacity isn't limited to athletic performance; it extends to everyday activities and overall vitality.

The cardiovascular system also benefits significantly from enhanced cellular energy production. The heart, with its constant energy demands, functions more efficiently when cellular energy production is optimized[64 45 20]. This improvement in cardiac energy metabolism can contribute to better overall cardiovascular health and function.

Systemic benefits also extend to the immune system. Immune cells require significant energy for proper function, and enhanced cellular energy production supports more efficient immune responses[64 45 20]. This improvement in immune function can contribute to better overall health and resilience.

The metabolic benefits of enhanced cellular energy production create a ripple effect throughout the body. Improved energy availability supports better hormone production, enhanced detoxification processes, and more efficient cellular repair mechanisms[64 20]. These improvements contribute to better overall health and function across multiple body systems.

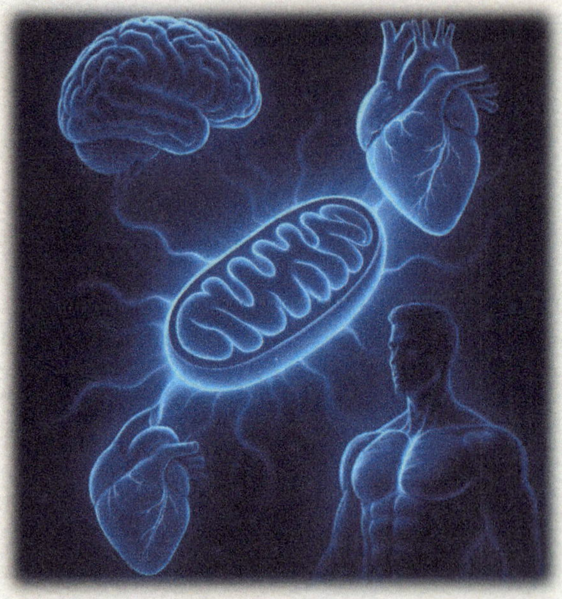

Perhaps most remarkably, the systemic benefits of methylene blue's energy enhancement appear to be self-reinforcing. As cellular energy production improves, cells become more efficient at maintaining their function and repairing damage[64 45 20]. This enhanced cellular maintenance helps preserve the very mechanisms that methylene blue supports, creating a positive cycle of improved health and function.

When implementing methylene blue for systemic energy enhancement, proper dosing becomes crucial. Research indicates that doses between 0.5 and 4 mg/kg body weight are most effective for optimizing cellular energy production without risking inhibitory effects[45 20]. This typically translates to daily doses of 4-30 mg for most adults.

Protocol Summary for Systemic Energy Enhancement:

- Initial dose: 4-8 mg daily
- Therapeutic range: 4-30 mg daily
- Optimal timing: Morning administration
- Duration: Ongoing with periodic assessment
- Quality requirement: Pharmaceutical-grade (USP) methylene blue
- Regular monitoring of response and adjustment as needed
- Contraindications: G6PD deficiency, serotonergic medications

By understanding the progression from cellular to systemic benefits, we can better appreciate the potential of methylene blue as a comprehensive energy enhancement compound. Its unique ability to optimize energy production while protecting cellular function makes it a valuable tool for supporting overall health and vitality.

Practical Applications for Fatigue and Energy Management

The application of methylene blue for fatigue and energy management represents one of its most promising therapeutic uses, particularly given the compound's unique ability to enhance mitochondrial function at the cellular level. Understanding how to implement methylene blue for energy enhancement effectively requires careful consideration of both dosing protocols and individual factors that may influence its effectiveness.

The scientific basis for using methylene blue in fatigue management stems from its direct impact on mitochondrial dysfunction, which is increasingly recognized as a central factor in various types of fatigue, including chronic fatigue and post-viral syndromes. Research has demonstrated that when mitochondrial efficiency declines, cells struggle to meet their energy demands, leading to persistent fatigue, brain fog, and impaired recovery[66 58].

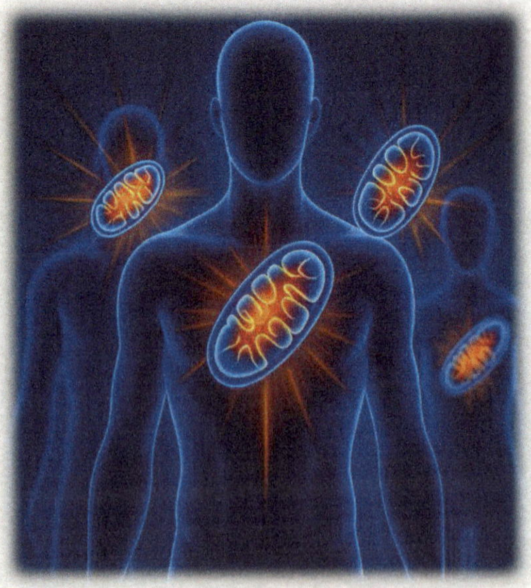

Methylene blue's mechanism of action in addressing fatigue operates through multiple complementary pathways. As a mitochondrial electron carrier, it enhances cellular respiration and ATP production, directly addressing energy deficits at their source[65 66]. Unlike conventional stimulants that provide temporary energy boosts, methylene blue supports sustainable cellular energy metabolism[68] while simultaneously reducing oxidative stress, a common feature in fatigue-related disorders[66].

The practical implementation of methylene blue for fatigue management typically involves several key considerations. First, dosing should start conservatively, usually between 0.5 and 4 mg/kg body weight, as higher doses may actually inhibit energy production. Morning administration often proves most effective, aligning with natural circadian rhythms and daily energy demands.

Clinical applications have shown particular promise in several areas of fatigue management. For individuals dealing with post-viral fatigue or recovery from chronic infections, methylene blue's ability to enhance mitochondrial function can provide crucial support for cellular energy production[65]. Additionally, its neuroprotective properties may help address the cognitive symptoms often associated with fatigue syndromes[65 58].

Safety considerations remain paramount when implementing methylene blue for the management of fatigue. While it has a well-established safety profile and appears on the World Health Organization's list of essential medications[65], certain precautions must be observed. Individuals taking serotonergic medications should exercise particular caution due to potential interactions, and those with G6PD deficiency should avoid use entirely[58].

Optimal results often emerge from a systematic approach to implementation. This includes:

- Starting with low doses (4-8 mg daily)
- Monitoring response and adjusting gradually as needed
- Maintaining consistent timing of administration
- Ensuring proper hydration
- Using pharmaceutical-grade methylene blue
- Regular assessment of effectiveness

The enhancement of cellular energy through methylene blue supplementation can lead to several systemic benefits that directly impact fatigue management:

- Improved cognitive clarity and reduced brain fog [65 58]

- Enhanced physical endurance and recovery[66]
- Better sleep quality
- Reduced oxidative stress[66 58]
- Improved cellular repair mechanisms

Current research suggests that the effectiveness of methylene blue for fatigue management may be further enhanced when combined with other supportive therapies. Some practitioners report success in combining methylene blue with normobaric hyperoxia or cold therapy[67], although more research is needed to understand these synergistic effects fully.

Protocol Summary for Fatigue Management:

- Initial dose: 4-8 mg daily
- Therapeutic range: 4-30 mg daily
- Optimal timing: Morning administration
- Duration: Ongoing with periodic assessment
- Quality requirement: Pharmaceutical-grade (USP) methylene blue

- Monitoring: Regular assessment of energy levels and cognitive function
- Contraindications: G6PD deficiency, serotonergic medications

While the current evidence base for methylene blue in fatigue management is promising, it's essential to note that most supporting data come from preclinical studies and clinical observations rather than large-scale, randomized controlled trials[67 58]. However, its well-established safety profile and mechanism of action make it a compelling option for those seeking to address persistent fatigue through cellular energy optimization.

The future of methylene blue in fatigue management appears promising, with ongoing research investigating optimal protocols and potential synergistic combinations with other therapies[67]. As our understanding of mitochondrial dysfunction in fatigue conditions continues to evolve, methylene blue's role as a therapeutic tool for energy enhancement may become increasingly significant.

Practical implementation should always begin with careful consideration of individual factors and potential contraindications. Working with a healthcare provider familiar with methylene blue protocols can help ensure the safe and effective use of this treatment, while maximizing its potential benefits for managing fatigue and enhancing energy.

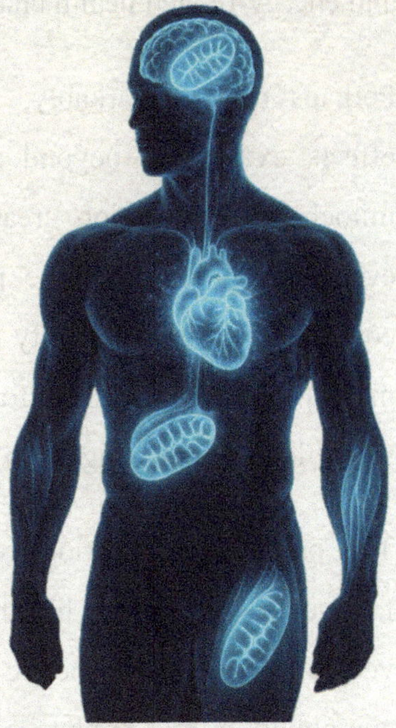

As we conclude our exploration of methylene blue's remarkable effects on cellular energy production and mitochondrial function, it's clear that this versatile molecule holds tremendous potential for supporting health and vitality at the most fundamental level. Throughout this chapter, we've uncovered how methylene blue serves as a unique alternative electron carrier, enhancing mitochondrial function while simultaneously protecting cells from oxidative damage.

The journey through cellular energetics has revealed several key insights about methylene blue's therapeutic potential. We've seen how it can increase ATP production by up to 30% while reducing harmful reactive oxygen species, creating a dual benefit that sets it apart from conventional supplements. Its ability to bypass compromised elements of the electron transport chain while supporting overall mitochondrial function makes it particularly valuable for addressing age-related decline and energy-related health challenges.

Perhaps most remarkably, we've discovered how methylene blue's effects extend far beyond simple energy enhancement. Optimizing mitochondrial function creates a cascade of benefits that influence everything from cognitive performance to physical endurance. The compound's unique ability to cross the blood-brain barrier while maintaining its electron transport capabilities makes it especially valuable for supporting brain health and mental clarity.

The practical applications we've explored ranging from addressing fatigue to supporting healthy aging—demonstrate methylene blue's versatility as a therapeutic tool. However, as with any powerful compound, proper implementation is crucial. The importance of proper dosing cannot be overstated, as research consistently shows that low doses (0.5-4 mg/kg) provide optimal benefits, while higher doses may actually inhibit cellular function.

Moving forward, it's essential to remember several key points about methylene blue's role in cellular energy production:

- The power of methylene blue lies in its ability to optimize rather than stimulate energy production

- Proper dosing is crucial - lower doses (4-30 mg daily for most adults) typically provide optimal benefits
- Quality matters - using pharmaceutical-grade methylene blue ensures safety and efficacy
- Individual responses may vary, making careful monitoring and adjustment important
- Some individuals, particularly those with G6PD deficiency or taking serotonergic medications, should avoid the use of methylene blue use

As we move into methylene blue's broader health benefits, remember that its power begins at the cellular level. By optimizing mitochondrial function and energy production, it sets off a cascade of effects that influence nearly every aspect of health and vitality.

Methylene blue's dual role enhancing cellular energy while protecting against oxidative stress, makes it a unique and valuable tool for advancing optimal health. When applied with understanding, it supports cellular function in ways that surpass simple stimulation or supplementation.

Armed with this knowledge, you can approach methylene blue with precision, whether your goal is to address specific conditions or elevate overall wellness.

In the next chapter, we'll translate these cellular mechanisms into ten concrete health benefits, connecting theory to practice and deepening our understanding of methylene blue's full therapeutic potential.

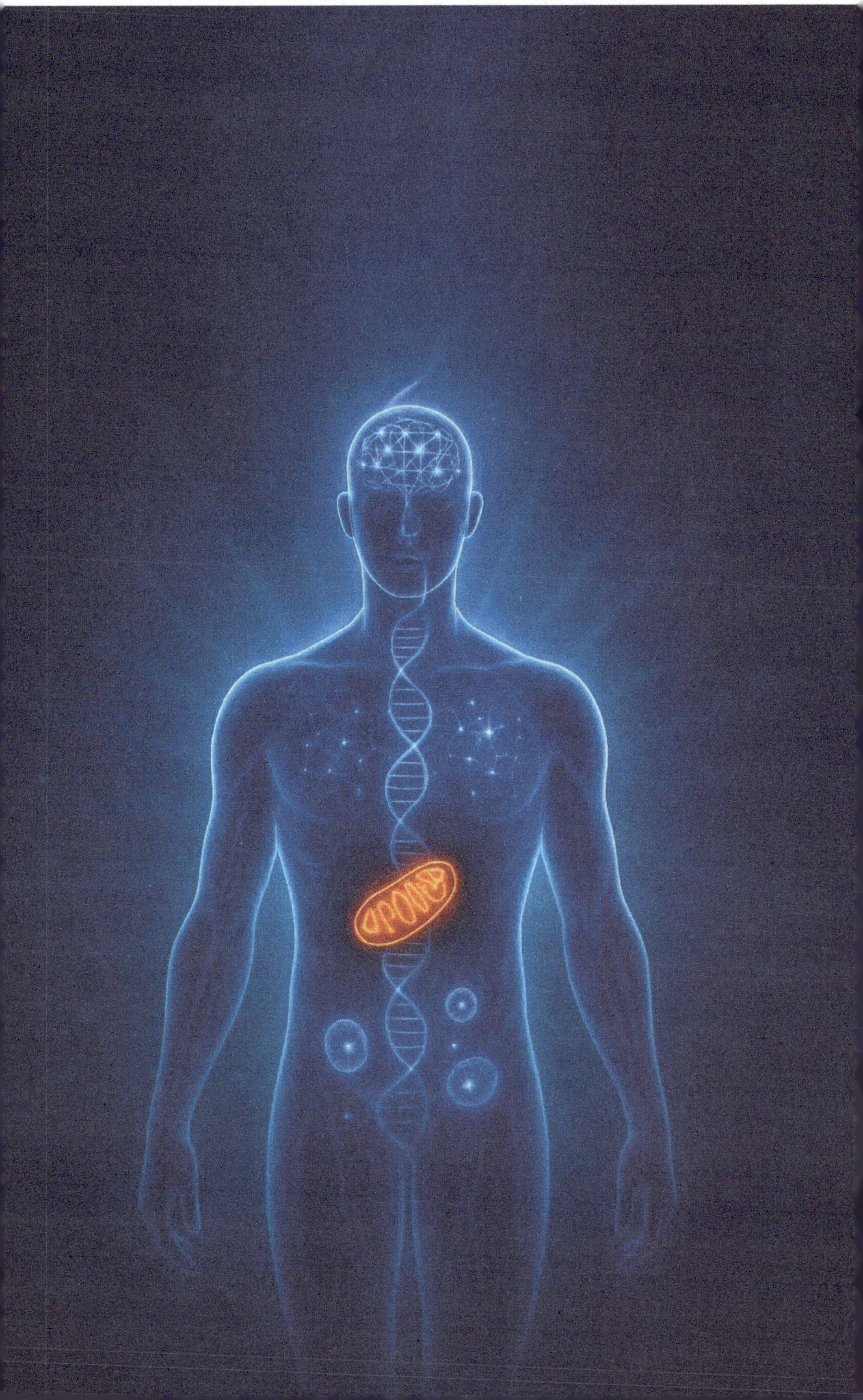

CHAPTER 3

TEN TRANSFORMATIVE BENEFITS: FROM BRAIN HEALTH TO CELLULAR REGENERATION

The human body is an intricate symphony of biological processes, each essential to maintaining health and vitality. Methylene blue acts as a master conductor in this orchestra, enhancing cellular energy production and reducing oxidative stress across multiple systems. This remarkable molecule influences a wide range of physiological functions, making it one of the most fascinating compounds in modern therapeutic science.

In this chapter, we'll explore ten transformative benefits of methylene blue, from boosting brain function to promoting cellular regeneration. Each benefit reveals how this compound supports optimal health and wellness, offering insight into how it may serve your individual goals.

What sets methylene blue apart is its ability to cross the blood-brain barrier and directly influence neural tissue. Combined with its potent antioxidant effects and role in energy metabolism, this property underlies its diverse therapeutic potential.

As we examine each benefit, we'll uncover the mechanisms behind methylene blue's impact, how it enhances cognition, supports cellular repair, and strengthens overall physiological performance.

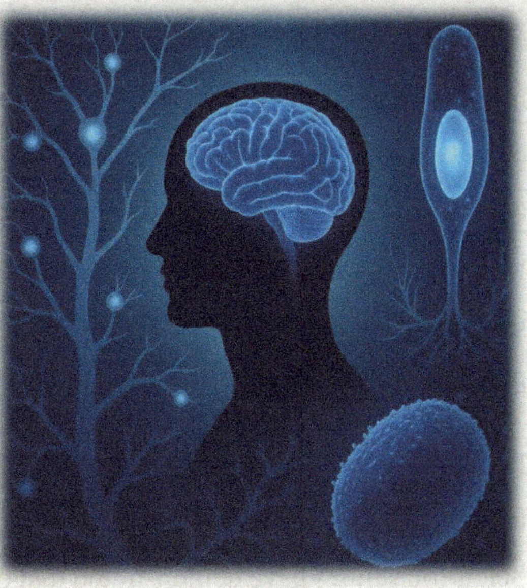

Its unique dual action—working at the microscopic cellular level while producing system-wide effects explains why methylene blue continues to draw attention in research and clinical practice.

By the end of this exploration, you'll see how this versatile compound promotes mental clarity, cellular health, and longevity, building upon the foundation of cellular optimization established in previous chapters.

Cognitive Enhancement and Memory Support

One of methylene blue's most remarkable capabilities lies in its ability to enhance cognitive function and support memory processes through multiple mechanisms. At the cellular level, this versatile molecule acts as an electron cycler in the mitochondrial electron transport chain, optimizing energy production specifically in neural tissues[70] [20]. This enhanced cellular energy availability provides the foundation for improved cognitive performance and memory consolidation.

The cognitive benefits of methylene blue stem primarily from its unique ability to cross the blood-brain barrier and directly influence neural metabolism. Research has shown that methylene blue increases the activity of cytochrome oxidase, a crucial enzyme in cellular respiration, resulting in a 30-70% increase in brain energy production[20]. This increase in neural energy availability directly translates to enhanced memory formation, improved attention, and better overall cognitive performance.

Particularly noteworthy is methylene blue's hormetic dose-response, meaning its cognitive benefits are most pronounced at low doses[70] [20]. Scientific studies have demonstrated that optimal cognitive enhancement occurs within a specific dosage range, typically 0.5-4 mg/kg, in research settings[20]. Beyond this range, the benefits may diminish or even reverse, underscoring the importance of adhering to proper dosing protocols.

The compound's neuroprotective properties extend beyond immediate cognitive enhancement. As a potent antioxidant, methylene blue helps shield neurons from oxidative damage, a common factor in age-related cognitive decline[70] [20]. By reducing reactive oxygen species and supporting cellular repair mechanisms, it helps maintain optimal brain function over time.

Human research has provided compelling evidence for methylene blue's cognitive benefits. Studies using functional MRI have shown that even a single dose can increase activity in brain regions responsible for short-term memory and attention, resulting in measurable improvements in memory retrieval[71]. These findings are supported by extensive laboratory research demonstrating enhanced long-term contextual memory and improved memory consolidation[71 20].

At the molecular level, methylene blue activates nuclear respiratory factors that promote the expression of mitochondrial enzymes[20]. This activation is particularly beneficial during periods of intense neural activity, such as learning and the formation of new synaptic connections. The increased metabolic support during these critical periods enhances the brain's ability to form and maintain new memories.

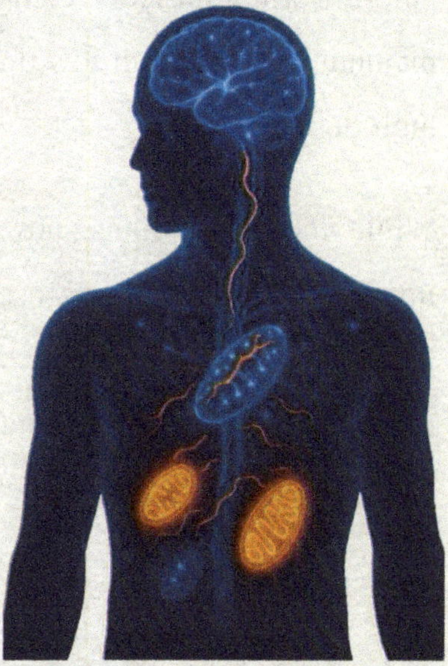

When considering methylene blue for cognitive enhancement, it's essential to note potential interactions with certain medications, particularly those affecting serotonin levels. Individuals taking SSRIs or other serotonergic medications should consult healthcare providers before using methylene blue, as combining these substances may lead to adverse effects.

The cognitive benefits of methylene blue are particularly relevant for addressing age-related cognitive decline and neurodegenerative conditions. Research suggests that its neuroprotective properties may help maintain cognitive function in aging populations[69 72], though long-term studies are still ongoing to understand its potential in this area fully.

Practical implementation of methylene blue for cognitive enhancement requires careful attention to timing and dosage. For optimal results, administration should align with periods of cognitive demand, such as before learning tasks or complex problem-solving activities. However, maintaining consistent low doses appears more beneficial than sporadic high-dose usage.

While methylene blue shows promise as a cognitive enhancer, it's important to approach its use as part of a comprehensive strategy for brain health. Combining methylene blue supplementation with proper nutrition, regular exercise, and adequate sleep can maximize its cognitive benefits while supporting overall brain function.

Neuroprotective Properties and Brain Health

Methylene blue's remarkable neuroprotective properties stem from its unique ability to enhance brain health through multiple pathways. At the cellular level, this versatile molecule acts as a powerful defender of neural tissue, protecting brain cells from damage while optimizing their function. Research has demonstrated that methylene blue's neuroprotective effects are particularly valuable in addressing various forms of neurodegeneration and supporting overall brain health.

One of methylene blue's primary neuroprotective mechanisms involves its ability to reroute electron flow within neurons. When certain parts of the cellular energy production system become damaged or compromised, methylene blue can effectively bypass these problem areas, ensuring continued ATP production[20]. This capability is crucial for maintaining neural health, as neurons require a constant energy supply to function properly.

The compound's antioxidant properties play a vital role in its neuroprotective effects. By accepting stray electrons, methylene blue prevents the formation of harmful reactive oxygen species (ROS) that can damage DNA, proteins, and cellular membranes[20]. This protection is particularly crucial in the brain, where oxidative stress can lead to accelerated aging and neurodegeneration.

Methylene blue's ability to enhance oxygen utilization in neural tissue represents another key aspect of its neuroprotective properties. Through its unique cycling between oxidized and reduced states, the compound supports essential cellular functions, including synaptic signaling and calcium buffering[20]. This optimization of cellular respiration helps maintain healthy brain function even under challenging conditions.

Research has shown promising results regarding the potential of methylene blue in addressing various neurodegenerative conditions. Studies indicate that the compound may help prevent neuronal damage and potentially alter disease progression in models of conditions such as Alzheimer's and Parkinson's disease[20 63]. Its ability to limit toxic protein aggregation, a common feature in many neurodegenerative disorders, makes it particularly interesting for therapeutic applications[20].

The compound's role in mitigating neuroinflammation adds another layer to its neuroprotective capabilities. Chronic inflammation in the brain is a common pathological feature across various neurodegenerative disorders[63], and methylene blue's anti-inflammatory properties may help address this underlying factor in brain health deterioration.

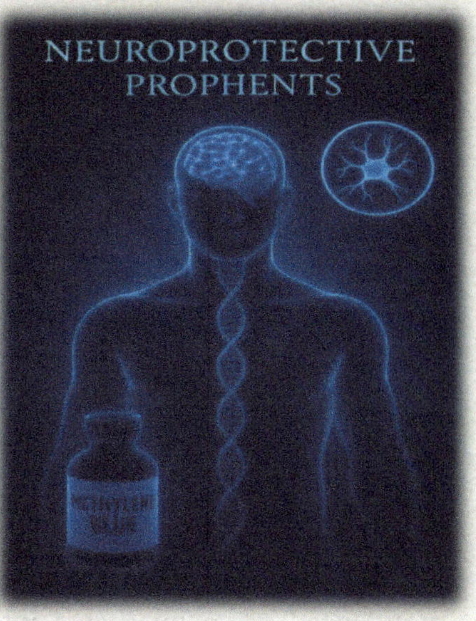

When considering methylene blue for brain health, it's essential to note that its effects appear to be dose-dependent. Research suggests that lower doses may be more effective for neuroprotection, as they allow the compound to work optimally without overwhelming cellular systems. This understanding has important implications for therapeutic applications.

The combination of methylene blue with other interventions, such as near-infrared light therapy, has shown promise in enhancing neuroprotective effects. Both approaches target mitochondrial respiration, potentially creating synergistic benefits for energy metabolism and neuronal survival[50]. However, any combination therapy should be approached with careful consideration and professional guidance.

For those interested in implementing methylene blue for brain health, it's crucial to maintain consistent, appropriate dosing rather than sporadic high-dose usage. Regular, low-dose administration appears to provide the most beneficial neuroprotective effects while minimizing the risk of adverse reactions.

While the research supporting methylene blue's neuroprotective properties is compelling, it's important to approach its use as part of a comprehensive brain health strategy. This includes maintaining a proper diet, engaging in regular exercise, getting adequate sleep, and practicing effective stress management. The compound's benefits are most pronounced when integrated into a holistic approach to brain health maintenance.

Mitochondrial Function and Energy Production

At the heart of methylene blue's remarkable therapeutic potential lies its profound impact on mitochondrial function and cellular energy production. These microscopic powerhouses within our cells are responsible for generating the energy currency known as ATP (adenosine triphosphate), which fuels virtually every biological process in the body. Methylene blue's unique ability to enhance mitochondrial efficiency makes it a powerful tool for optimizing cellular energy production.[58 49]

Methylene blue serves as an electron shuttle in the mitochondrial electron transport chain (ETC), thereby enhancing the efficiency of cellular respiration. By accepting electrons and transferring them through the ETC, methylene blue helps bypass potential blockages or inefficiencies in this vital energy-producing pathway. This process results in increased ATP production and improved cellular energy availability.[20 49]

One of methylene blue's most significant advantages is its ability to serve as a renewable antioxidant within the mitochondria. Unlike traditional antioxidants that become depleted after neutralizing free radicals, methylene blue can cycle between its oxidized and reduced forms, providing continuous protection against oxidative stress while supporting energy production[20]. This unique characteristic makes it particularly valuable for maintaining long-term mitochondrial health.

Research has demonstrated that methylene blue can increase cellular oxygen consumption and ATP production by 30-70% under optimal conditions[20]. This substantial enhancement in energy production has important implications for conditions characterized by mitochondrial dysfunction or energy deficits. The compound's ability to improve mitochondrial efficiency becomes especially crucial in high-energy-demanding tissues such as the brain and heart.

Methylene blue's support of mitochondrial function extends beyond simple energy production. Improving the efficiency of the electron transport chain helps reduce the production of harmful reactive oxygen species (ROS), which are byproducts of cellular respiration that are damaging to cells[58 49]. This dual action of enhancing energy production while limiting oxidative stress creates a powerful synergistic effect for cellular health.

The compound's interaction with mitochondria follows a hormetic dose response, meaning its benefits are most pronounced within a specific dosage range. Low to moderate doses typically provide optimal support for mitochondrial function, while excessive doses may actually impair energy production. This understanding underscores the importance of adhering to proper dosing protocols when utilizing methylene blue for mitochondrial support.

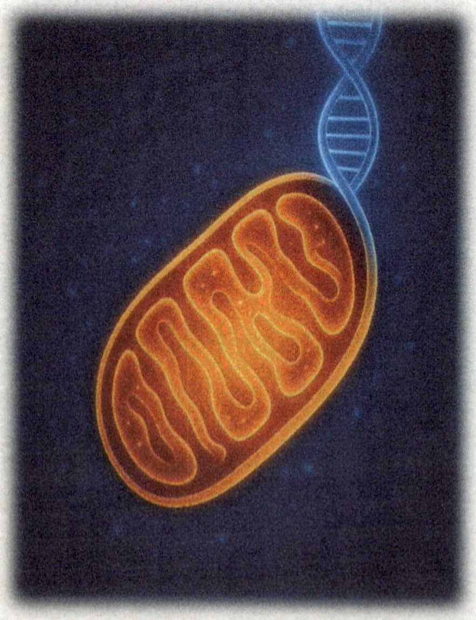

For those interested in implementing methylene blue for

mitochondrial support, timing can be crucial. Administration is often most beneficial during periods of high energy demand or when cellular energy production may be compromised. However, it's essential to start with low doses and gradually adjust based on individual response while monitoring for any potential interactions with existing medications.

The benefits of enhanced mitochondrial function extend throughout the body, influencing everything from cognitive performance to physical endurance. Improved energy production at the cellular level can lead to better mental clarity, increased physical stamina, and enhanced overall vitality[20 49]. This systemic impact makes methylene blue a valuable tool for supporting general health and wellness.

When considering methylene blue for mitochondrial support, it's essential to note that its effects can be enhanced by incorporating proper lifestyle factors. Adequate nutrition, regular exercise, and stress management all play crucial roles in supporting mitochondrial health. Methylene blue is most effective when used as part of a comprehensive approach to cellular health, rather than as a standalone intervention.

While the research supporting methylene blue's role in mitochondrial function is compelling, ongoing studies continue to reveal new aspects of its mechanism of action and potential applications. The compound's ability to optimize cellular energy production while providing antioxidant protection makes it a promising therapeutic agent for various conditions associated with mitochondrial dysfunction[58] [20]. As our understanding of methylene blue's effects on cellular energy production continues to grow, its importance in supporting mitochondrial health becomes increasingly evident.

Antimicrobial and Immune System Support

Methylene blue's remarkable antimicrobial properties and immune system support capabilities make it a powerful therapeutic agent in fighting infections and maintaining overall health[73] [74] [75] [76] [77]. This versatile compound works through multiple mechanisms to combat pathogens while potentially supporting the body's natural defense systems. Understanding these properties helps explain why methylene blue has remained a valuable tool in medical applications for over a century.

At its core, methylene blue acts as a potent antimicrobial agent through several distinct mechanisms. When introduced to microbial cells, it generates reactive oxygen species (ROS) that cause oxidative damage to essential cellular components, leading to the death of the microbial cells[73]. This process is particularly effective because methylene blue can penetrate cellular membranes and target specific biological processes within harmful microorganisms.

One of methylene blue's most significant advantages is its broad-spectrum activity against various pathogens. Research has demonstrated its effectiveness against numerous bacteria, including challenging strains such as Staphylococcus aureus and Escherichia coli[75 76]. The compound also shows promise against certain fungal species such as Candida albicans[75], making it a versatile antimicrobial agent.

Methylene blue's ability to disrupt biofilms represents another crucial aspect of its antimicrobial action. Biofilms are protective layers that bacteria create to shield themselves from antibiotics and other treatments. By breaking down these defensive structures, methylene blue not only directly fights infection but also enhances the effectiveness of other antimicrobial therapies[74].

In clinical applications, methylene blue has shown particular promise when used in combination with photodynamic therapy (MB-PDT). When exposed to red light, the antimicrobial properties of methylene blue are significantly enhanced, creating a powerful treatment option for localized infections. This approach has proven especially valuable in addressing drug-resistant bacterial strains[76].

The compound's role in immune system support, while still being actively researched, appears to work through multiple pathways. By controlling infection and reducing pathogen-induced inflammation, methylene blue helps create an environment that supports optimal immune function[73]

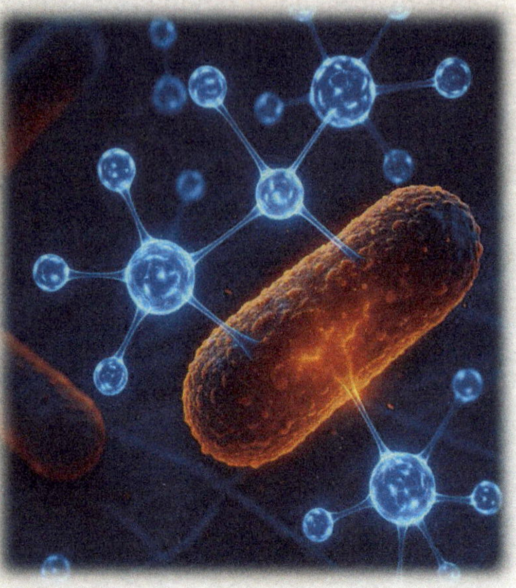

[74]. Its ability to modulate oxidative stress also contributes to its potential immune-supporting properties.

Laboratory studies have provided compelling evidence for methylene blue's antimicrobial efficacy. Research has shown that even at relatively low concentrations (0.05% to 0.1%), methylene blue can significantly reduce the colony-forming units of various pathogenic bacteria[75]. These findings support the practical application of this approach in both clinical and laboratory settings.

When considering methylene blue for antimicrobial purposes, it is crucial to use the proper concentration and application methods. The compound's effectiveness often depends on factors such as exposure time, concentration, and the specific type of pathogen being targeted.

This understanding helps guide the development of appropriate therapeutic protocols and applications.

Methylene blue's stability and safety profile make it particularly valuable in medical applications. Unlike some traditional disinfectants that may degrade quickly or pose handling risks, methylene blue remains stable and is generally safe when used appropriately[77]. This characteristic has contributed to its enduring role in medical and laboratory settings.

For those interested in implementing methylene blue for its antimicrobial properties, it's essential to understand proper protocols and potential interactions. While the compound exhibits remarkable versatility in combating infections, its use should be approached with careful consideration of individual circumstances and under the guidance of a qualified medical professional.

The synergistic potential of methylene blue with conventional antibiotics represents an exciting frontier in antimicrobial therapy. Research suggests that combining methylene blue with certain antibiotics may enhance their effectiveness, particularly against resistant strains[73 74 76]. This synergy offers promising possibilities for addressing the growing challenge of antibiotic resistance.

As research continues to unveil new aspects of methylene blue's antimicrobial and immune-supporting properties, its importance in therapeutic applications continues to grow. The compound's ability to combat infection while potentially supporting immune function makes it a valuable tool in the modern medical arsenal, particularly in an era of increasing antimicrobial resistance.

Cellular Repair and Regeneration Mechanisms

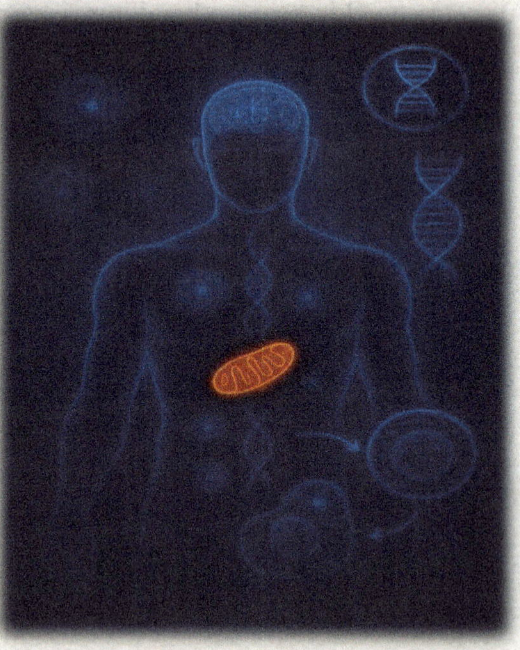

Methylene blue's remarkable ability to support cellular repair and regeneration represents one of its most fascinating therapeutic properties. At the cellular level, this versatile molecule acts through multiple pathways to enhance the body's natural repair mechanisms while protecting against further damage[45 78 20]. Understanding these processes reveals why methylene blue has emerged as a powerful tool for supporting cellular health and longevity.

At its core, methylene blue enhances cellular repair by optimizing mitochondrial function and ATP production. Research has shown that methylene blue can serve as an electron shuttle within mitochondria, particularly effective when the electron transport chain is damaged or inefficient. In its reduced form, it can donate electrons directly to cytochrome c or other downstream components, effectively bypassing blockages and sustaining ATP synthesis[20 78 45]. This capability ensures that cells maintain the energy needed for repair and regeneration, even under stressful conditions.

One of methylene blue's most significant contributions to cellular repair comes through its potent antioxidant properties. Studies have demonstrated that methylene blue can reduce intracellular oxidant levels by up to 28%, providing crucial protection for DNA, proteins, and cellular membranes from oxidative damage[78 79 54]. This protection is particularly valuable as oxidative stress is a major contributor to cellular aging and dysfunction.

The compound's ability to stimulate mitochondrial biogenesis represents another crucial mechanism supporting cellular repair. Research has shown that methylene blue induces the expression of key regulators, such as PGC1-α and SURF1, which control mitochondrial biogenesis and complex IV assembly[79]. This increased mitochondrial capacity enhances the cell's ability to generate energy needed for repair processes.

Methylene blue also plays a vital role in activating cellular defense pathways. Through its interaction with the Keap1/Nrf2 pathway, a central cellular defense mechanism, methylene blue helps upregulate antioxidant response elements[79]. This activation enhances the cell's natural ability to detoxify and repair itself, creating a more robust cellular defense system.

Notably, methylene blue's impact on cellular senescence and aging is particularly noteworthy. Research has demonstrated that methylene blue treatment can delay cellular aging by slowing telomere erosion, a key marker of cellular lifespan[79]. Studies indicate its anti-senescence effect is approximately eight times more potent than AICAR[79], another known activator of cellular repair pathways.

The compound's enhancement of autophagy, the process by which cells remove and recycle damaged components, provides another crucial mechanism for cellular repair80. This "cellular cleanup" process is essential for maintaining healthy cellular function and preventing the accumulation of damaged cellular components that can lead to dysfunction and disease.

When implementing methylene blue for cellular repair and regeneration, proper dosing is crucial. Research suggests that lower doses often prove most effective for supporting cellular repair mechanisms, as they allow the compound to work optimally without overwhelming cellular systems[20 45]. This understanding has important implications for therapeutic applications.

It's important to note that the cellular repair benefits of methylene blue are most pronounced when combined with proper lifestyle factors. Adequate nutrition, regular exercise, and stress management all play crucial roles in supporting cellular repair processes. Methylene blue is most effective when used as part of a comprehensive approach to cellular health, rather than as a standalone intervention.

While the research supporting methylene blue's role in cellular repair and regeneration is compelling, ongoing studies continue to reveal new aspects of its mechanism of action. The compound's ability to support multiple repair pathways while providing antioxidant protection makes it a promising therapeutic agent for various conditions associated with cellular damage and aging[78 20 79 45 80 53 54]. As our understanding of methylene blue's effects on cellular repair continues to grow, its importance in supporting cellular health becomes increasingly evident.

Cardiovascular Health Benefits

Methylene blue's cardiovascular benefits represent one of its most significant therapeutic applications, particularly in critical care and surgical settings[81 82 83]. This remarkable compound influences cardiovascular health through multiple mechanisms, most notably by interacting with nitric oxide signaling pathways and exhibiting potent antioxidant properties[81 82 83]. Understanding these mechanisms reveals why methylene blue has become an increasingly valuable tool in cardiovascular medicine.

At the molecular level, methylene blue acts as a selective inhibitor of soluble guanylate cyclase (sGC), thereby effectively modulating nitric

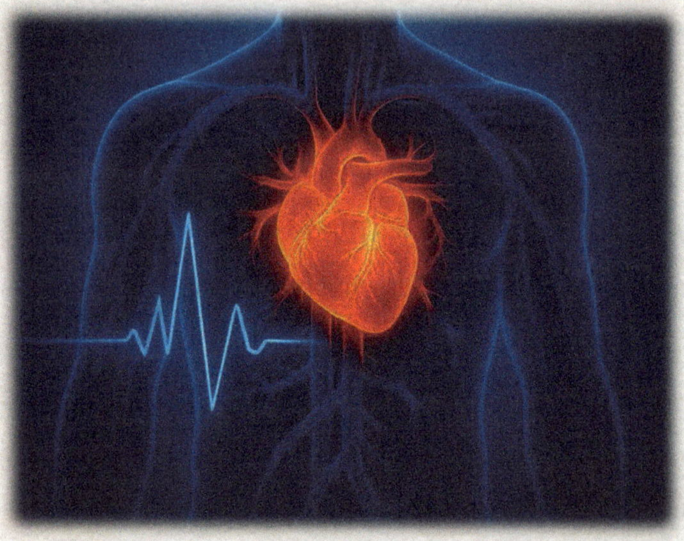

oxide-mediated vasodilation83. This action proves particularly beneficial in managing conditions characterized by excessive vasodilation, such as vasodilatory shock. Research has demonstrated that methylene blue can help restore vascular tone and improve blood pressure regulation when standard treatments prove insufficient[81 83].

One of methylene blue's most significant cardiovascular applications lies in its ability to support hemodynamic stability. Meta-analyses of clinical studies have shown that when administered alongside conventional vasopressors, methylene blue significantly reduces mortality rates in patients with vasodilatory shock. The data indicate an impressive odds ratio of 0.54 for mortality reduction, highlighting its potential life-saving capabilities in critical care settings[81].

The compound's role in protecting against ischemia-reperfusion injury represents another significant benefit of its cardiovascular effects. Laboratory research has demonstrated that methylene blue, when administered after ischemia but before reperfusion, significantly reduces the incidence of arrhythmias and conduction blocks[82]. This timing-dependent protection stems from its ability to mitigate oxidative stress and inflammation during the reperfusion phase[82].

Notably, methylene blue's application in post-cardiac surgery scenarios has demonstrated remarkable efficacy in managing vasoplegic syndrome. Clinical evidence indicates that early administration of methylene blue following cardiac surgery can improve hemodynamics, reduce vasopressor requirements, and potentially lower both mortality and renal failure rates[83].

The compound's cardiovascular benefits extend beyond acute care settings. Its antioxidant properties and ability to enhance mitochondrial function may provide long-term cardiovascular protection by reducing oxidative stress and supporting cellular energy production in cardiac tissue[82]. This dual action makes it particularly valuable for maintaining cardiovascular health.

When considering methylene blue for cardiovascular applications, proper dosing and timing are crucial. Research indicates that the compound's effects are dose-dependent, with optimal benefits typically achieved at moderate doses. However, timing proves especially critical in certain applications, such as ischemia-reperfusion scenarios, where administration before ischemia could potentially increase risks[82].

Safety considerations in cardiovascular applications remain paramount. While methylene blue demonstrates an impressive safety profile, healthcare providers should monitor for rare complications such as acute pulmonary hypertension[81 83]. Additionally, potential interactions with certain medications, particularly those affecting serotonin levels, require careful consideration.

The compound's ability to improve tissue perfusion and oxygen metabolism, as evidenced by decreased lactate levels in clinical studies, suggests broader implications for cardiovascular health[81]. This improvement in cellular energetics may contribute to better overall cardiovascular function and recovery in various clinical scenarios.

For those considering methylene blue's cardiovascular applications, it's essential to understand that its benefits are most pronounced when integrated into comprehensive treatment protocols. While the compound shows remarkable promise in various cardiovascular applications, its use should always be guided by appropriate medical expertise and current clinical evidence[83].

Research continues to reveal new aspects of methylene blue's cardiovascular benefits, particularly in areas such as myocardial protection and vascular function[82 83]. As our understanding grows, so does the potential for expanding its therapeutic applications in cardiovascular medicine, making it an increasingly valuable tool in the medical arsenal for supporting heart health and vascular function.

Mood and Mental Health Support

Methylene blue's impact on mood and mental health represents one of its most promising therapeutic applications, supported by both historical use and modern research[84 64]. This versatile compound influences mental well-being through multiple mechanisms, particularly its effects on neurotransmitter regulation and mitochondrial function. Understanding these mechanisms reveals why methylene blue has become a valuable tool for promoting emotional balance and mental clarity.

At the molecular level, methylene blue acts as a monoamine oxidase (MAO) inhibitor, specifically targeting MAO-A. This action helps maintain optimal levels of crucial neurotransmitters, such as serotonin and dopamine, by slowing their breakdown in the brain[84 64]. Research has demonstrated that this mechanism contributes significantly to the compound's mood-stabilizing properties, particularly in cases of depression and anxiety.

One of methylene blue's most significant contributions to mental health comes through its ability to optimize mitochondrial function in neural tissue. Studies have shown that by acting as an alternative electron carrier in mitochondria, methylene blue enhances cellular energy production while reducing oxidative stress[84 85 64]. This dual action helps maintain optimal brain function and supports emotional resilience.

The compound's role in neurotransmitter regulation extends beyond simple MAO inhibition. Research indicates that methylene blue can enhance neurotransmitter signaling pathways, thereby supporting emotional stability, motivation, and focus[64]. This comprehensive effect on neural communication makes it particularly valuable for addressing various aspects of mood and mental health.

Particularly noteworthy is methylene blue's potential in bipolar disorder management. Clinical research has demonstrated its efficacy in both short- and long-term treatment, with the remarkable ability to improve mood without increasing the risk of manic episodes[84 86]. This characteristic sets it apart from many traditional antidepressants.

Dosing considerations prove crucial when using methylene blue for mood support. Studies indicate that lower doses (around 15 mg/day) often prove most effective, following a hormetic dose-response curve[86].

Higher doses may not necessarily provide additional benefits and could increase the risk of side effects.

Safety considerations are paramount when implementing methylene blue for mood support. The compound's MAO-inhibiting properties necessitate careful consideration of potential interactions with other medications, particularly those that affect serotonin levels[84 64]. Healthcare provider consultation is essential, especially for individuals taking SSRIs or other serotonergic medications.

The compound's cognitive-enhancing properties complement its mood-stabilizing effects. Research suggests that methylene blue can enhance memory and mental clarity, while also supporting emotional regulation[84]. This combination of cognitive and emotional benefits makes it particularly valuable for comprehensive mental health support.

When considering methylene blue for mood and mental health support, it's essential to understand that its benefits are most pronounced when integrated into a comprehensive approach to mental wellness. While the compound shows remarkable promise in various psychiatric applications, its effectiveness is enhanced when combined with proper nutrition, regular exercise, stress management, and professional support.

Ongoing research continues to unveil new aspects of methylene blue's effects on mood and mental health. The compound's ability to support multiple aspects of neural function while providing neuroprotective benefits makes it a promising therapeutic agent for various mental health conditions[84 86 64]. As our understanding grows, the role of methylene blue in supporting emotional well-being and mental clarity becomes increasingly evident.

Longevity and Anti-Aging Effects

Methylene blue's remarkable potential for promoting longevity and combating biological aging processes has garnered significant attention in recent scientific research[54 53]. This versatile compound works through multiple pathways to support cellular health and longevity, making it a promising candidate for anti-aging applications. Understanding these mechanisms reveals why methylene blue has emerged as a valuable tool in the pursuit of healthy aging.

At its core, methylene blue's anti-aging effects stem from its unique ability to enhance mitochondrial function. Research has demonstrated that methylene blue acts as an alternative electron carrier in the mitochondrial electron transport chain, facilitating more efficient ATP production while reducing the formation of harmful reactive oxygen species (ROS)[87 88 54]. This optimization of cellular energy production is crucial for maintaining tissue health and function throughout the aging process[87 88 53].

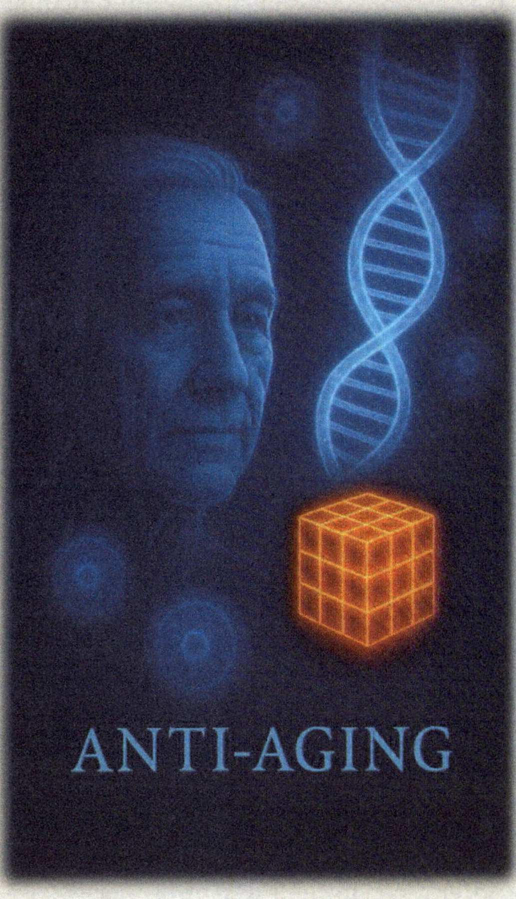

One of methylene blue's most significant contributions to longevity comes through its potent antioxidant properties. The compound's low redox potential enables it to efficiently cycle between oxidized and reduced forms, effectively scavenging ROS and breaking the cycle of mitochondrial damage and oxidative stress[54 53 90]. This protection against oxidative damage helps preserve cellular function and may slow the progression of age-related decline[87 53].

Particularly noteworthy is methylene blue's ability to delay cellular senescence - a key marker of biological aging. Research has shown that methylene blue can reduce the expression of p16, a biomarker of cellular aging, and delay senescence in skin fibroblasts[54 53]. Studies have even demonstrated its effectiveness in cells from patients with Hutchinson-Gilford progeria syndrome, a model of accelerated aging[54 53].

The compound's neuroprotective properties play a crucial role in its anti-aging effects. The brain is particularly susceptible to aging due to its high energy demands and sensitivity to oxidative stress[88 53 89 20]. Methylene blue helps protect neurons, reduces inflammation, and improves mitochondrial function in the central nervous system. Animal studies have revealed improved cognitive function and reduced neurodegeneration following methylene blue administration[88 89 20].

Research has shown promising results regarding the potential of methylene blue to extend cellular and organismal lifespan. Laboratory studies have demonstrated increased cellular lifespan and improved proliferation in cultured fibroblasts[54 53]. Additionally, female mice receiving methylene blue in their diet showed a 6% increase in lifespan, suggesting significant potential for organism-level anti-aging effects[54].

Methylene blue's impact on skin aging represents another fascinating aspect of its anti-aging properties. The compound has demonstrated remarkable abilities in delaying skin aging by protecting skin fibroblasts from oxidative stress, promoting healthy cell proliferation, and rescuing abnormal nuclear and mitochondrial features in premature aging models[54 90].

When considering methylene blue for anti-aging purposes, proper dosing is crucial. Research indicates that lower doses often prove most effective, following a hormetic dose-response curve. This understanding has important implications for therapeutic applications, as higher doses may not necessarily provide additional benefits and could increase the risk of side effects.

Safety considerations remain paramount when implementing methylene blue for longevity purposes. While the compound is FDA-approved for several medical uses and generally considered safe at low doses, potential interactions with certain medications, particularly SSRIs, require careful attention[87 53]. Professional guidance is essential when incorporating methylene blue into an anti-aging protocol.

The scientific evidence supporting the role of methylene blue in promoting longevity continues to grow. Its ability to target multiple aspects of cellular aging while providing broad-spectrum protection makes it a promising therapeutic agent for various age-related conditions[87 88 54 53 89 90 20]. As research advances, the importance of methylene blue in supporting healthy aging becomes increasingly evident, offering hope for those seeking to optimize their longevity potential through evidence-based interventions.

Oxidative Stress Reduction and Antioxidant Properties

Methylene blue's extraordinary antioxidant properties and ability to reduce oxidative stress represent some of its most powerful therapeutic benefits[20 52 91 53]. This remarkable molecule stands apart from conventional antioxidants due to its unique ability to cycle between oxidized and reduced states, effectively creating a renewable antioxidant system within cells[20 52]. Understanding these mechanisms reveals why methylene blue has become increasingly valuable in therapeutic applications targeting conditions related to oxidative stress.

At its core, methylene blue functions as a distinctive type of antioxidant that can be continuously recycled within cellular systems[20 52]. Unlike traditional antioxidants that become depleted after neutralizing free radicals, methylene blue maintains its antioxidant capacity through efficient redox cycling[20 52 91]. Research has demonstrated that this cycling ability allows methylene blue to provide sustained protection against oxidative damage while supporting cellular energy production.

One of methylene blue's most significant advantages lies in its direct interaction with mitochondrial function. By facilitating electron transfer in the electron transport chain, particularly through donations to cytochrome c, methylene blue helps optimize mitochondrial efficiency[20 91 92]. Studies have shown this optimization can increase mitochondrial oxygen consumption by up to 70% while boosting ATP production by approximately 30%[20]. This enhanced efficiency naturally reduces the formation of harmful reactive oxygen species (ROS) at their source.

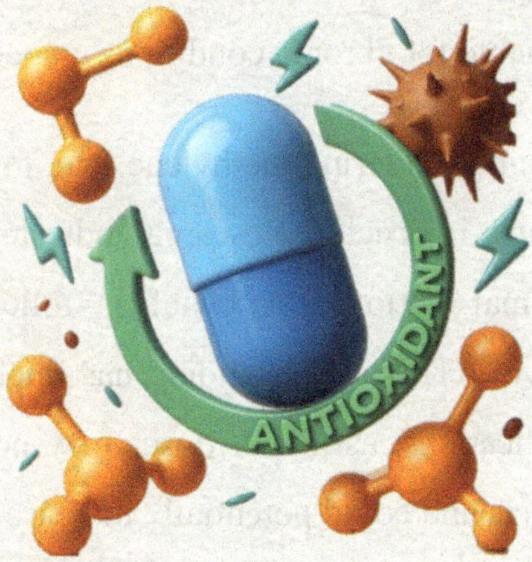

The compound's ability to target mitochondria sets it explicitly apart from conventional antioxidants. Methylene blue accumulates within mitochondria, where it can prevent ROS formation at its primary source rather than simply neutralizing existing free radicals[20 91]. This targeted approach offers more comprehensive protection against oxidative stress than traditional antioxidants, which may not reach these crucial cellular components.

Notably, methylene blue plays a crucial role in stabilizing cellular and mitochondrial structures. Research has shown that the compound helps maintain mitochondrial membrane integrity while supporting DNA repair mechanisms[52 91]. This dual action not only protects against immediate oxidative damage but also helps preserve long-term cellular health and function.

The antioxidant properties of methylene blue extend beyond simple ROS neutralization. Its unique molecular structure, featuring a delocalized π-electron system, contributes to its stability and ongoing antioxidant capacity[20]. This structural resilience enables methylene blue to maintain its protective effects over extended periods, making it particularly valuable for chronic conditions associated with oxidative stress.

When considering methylene blue for reducing oxidative stress, proper dosing is crucial. Research indicates that lower doses often provide optimal antioxidant benefits, following a hormetic dose-response curve[20]. This understanding has important implications for therapeutic applications, as higher doses may not necessarily enhance antioxidant effects and could potentially increase the risk of side effects.

The compound's ability to cross the blood-brain barrier while maintaining its antioxidant properties makes it particularly valuable for addressing oxidative stress in neural tissue[20 91 53]. This characteristic has led to increasing interest in methylene blue's potential applications for neurodegenerative conditions where oxidative stress plays a central role in disease progression.

Safety considerations remain paramount when using methylene blue due to its antioxidant properties. While the compound demonstrates an impressive safety profile at appropriate doses, potential interactions with certain medications require careful attention. Professional guidance proves essential when incorporating methylene blue into an antioxidant protocol, particularly for individuals taking medications that affect redox balance.

The scientific evidence supporting methylene blue's role in reducing oxidative stress continues to expand[20 52 91 53 54]. Its unique ability to provide renewable antioxidant protection while supporting mitochondrial function makes it a promising therapeutic agent for various conditions associated with oxidative stress. As research advances, the importance of methylene blue in supporting cellular health through antioxidant mechanisms becomes increasingly evident, offering hope for those seeking effective strategies to combat oxidative stress-related conditions.

As we conclude our exploration of methylene blue's ten transformative benefits, it's evident that this molecule offers far more than its origins as a textile dye suggest. From enhancing cognitive function and mitochondrial efficiency to supporting longevity and cardiovascular resilience, methylene blue proves to be a remarkably versatile therapeutic agent.

At the cellular level, it enhances mitochondrial performance, reduces oxidative stress, and supports essential biological processes. Its ability to cross the blood–brain barrier makes it especially valuable for cognitive enhancement and neuroprotection, while its antimicrobial and immunomodulatory properties further expand its therapeutic scope.

What distinguishes methylene blue is its role as a renewable antioxidant, cycling continuously between oxidized and reduced forms to provide sustained defense against oxidative damage. Combined with its mitochondrial optimization, this property positions it as a uniquely potent support for long-term vitality.

Its cardiovascular applications ranging from maintaining healthy blood pressure to protecting against ischemic injury, underscore its clinical importance. Meanwhile, its modulation of neurotransmitter systems and cellular energetics offers a natural avenue for supporting mood and emotional balance.

Throughout this chapter, we've stressed that methylene blue's benefits depend on proper dosing and respect for its hormetic nature: lower doses often yield the most therapeutic results. Understanding its pharmacology and potential interactions is crucial for safe, effective use.

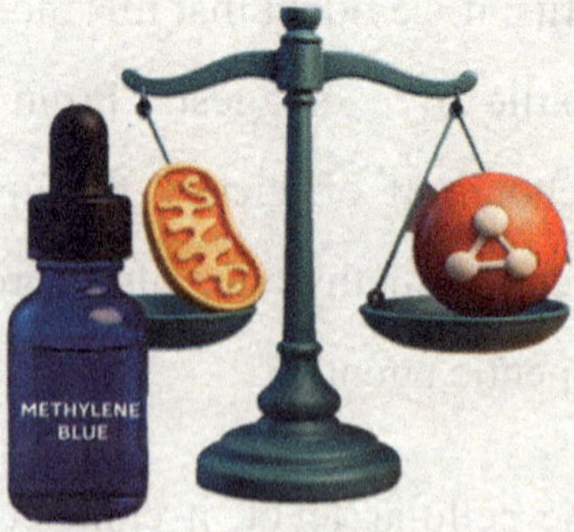

As research expands, methylene blue continues to reveal new potential in cellular repair, neuroprotection, and age-related disease. Integrating it within a broader foundation of nutrition, exercise, stress management, and restorative sleep amplifies its effects and promotes true systemic vitality.

In the next chapter, we'll move from principle to practice, covering protocols, dosing strategies, and safety guidelines to help you apply methylene blue effectively and responsibly.

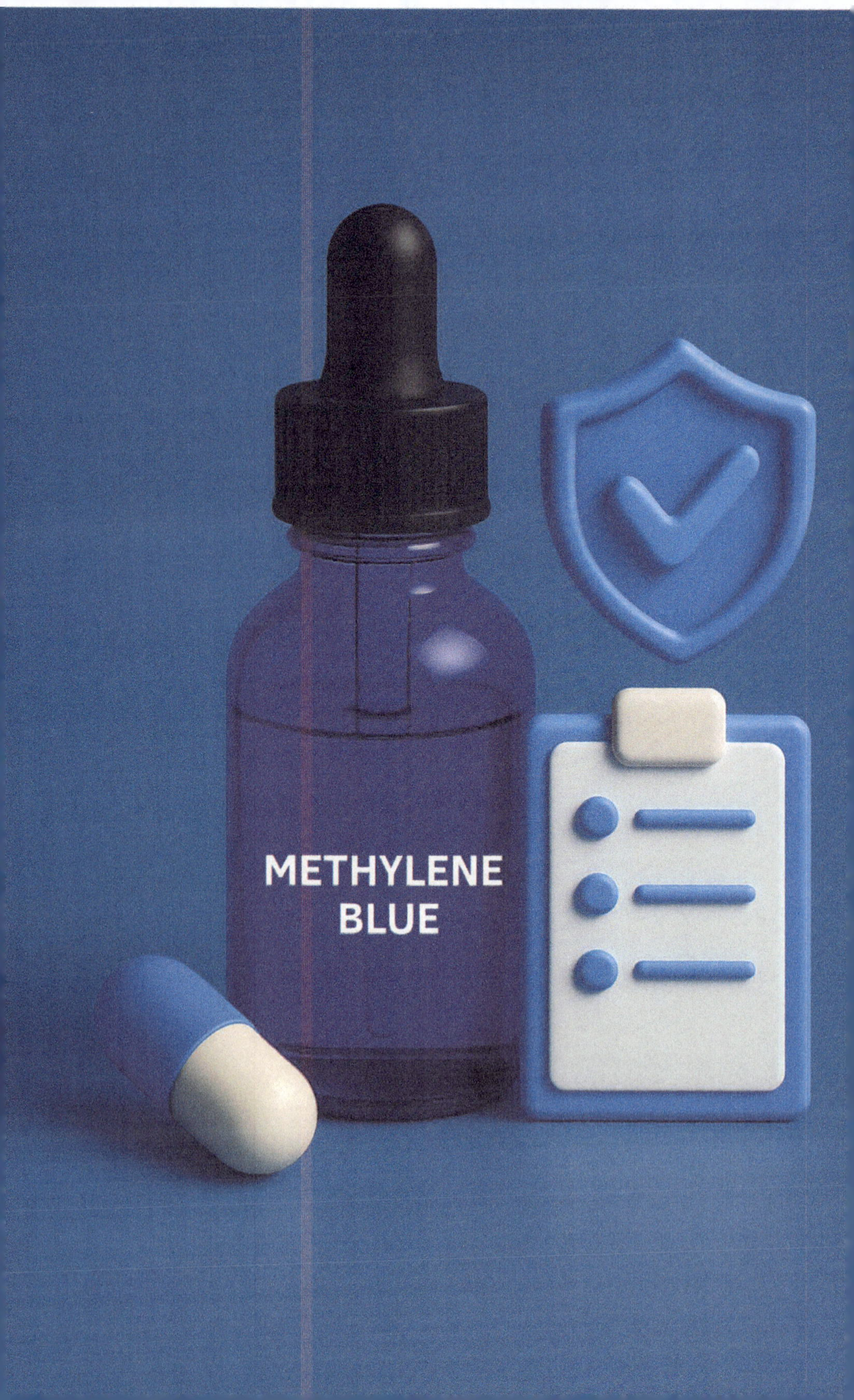
METHYLENE
BLUE

CHAPTER 4

THE PRACTICAL PROTOCOL: DOSING, SAFETY, AND STORAGE GUIDELINES

The journey from understanding the benefits of methylene blue to implementing it effectively requires meticulous attention to detail and adherence to established protocols. As a medical professional who has both administered and personally used methylene blue, I've learned that success lies in the precision of dosing, the adherence to safety guidelines, and the proper storage of this remarkable compound.

This chapter serves as your comprehensive guide to harnessing the therapeutic potential of methylene blue safely and effectively. Whether you're new to methylene blue supplementation or looking to optimize your current protocol, understanding proper dosing, safety considerations, and storage methods is crucial for achieving optimal results.

The science behind methylene blue dosing involves careful consideration of several factors, including body weight, intended therapeutic use, and individual sensitivity. While methylene blue has demonstrated an impressive safety profile when used correctly, precision in measurement and adherence to established guidelines are essential.

Proper storage and handling of methylene blue solutions are equally important aspects that can significantly impact their therapeutic effectiveness. Like many bioactive compounds, the potency of methylene blue can be affected by environmental factors, including light exposure, temperature fluctuations, and the type of storage container used.

In this chapter, we'll explore precise dosing protocols for various applications, examine critical safety considerations, including potential interactions with medications, and outline proper storage methods to maintain potency. You'll learn how to calculate appropriate doses based on your specific needs, understand the importance of timing and frequency of administration, and recognize signs of quality degradation.

By mastering these practical aspects of methylene blue use, you'll be better equipped to maximize its benefits while minimizing any potential risks. Let's begin by examining the fundamental principles of proper dosing and measurement, building a foundation for safe and effective methylene blue implementation.

Understanding Concentration Levels and Proper Measurement

Understanding the precise concentration of methylene blue solutions is fundamental to its safe and effective use. Whether you're using pharmaceutical or laboratory-grade methylene blue, knowing how to measure and verify concentration levels properly ensures you receive the intended therapeutic benefits while avoiding potential risks.

Methylene blue typically comes in two primary forms: as a crystalline powder that must be dissolved or as a pre-made solution. The concentration is usually expressed in milligrams per milliliter (mg/mL), milligrams per liter (mg/L), or as a percentage. For therapeutic use, common stock solutions are prepared at a concentration of 1% weight/volume (w/v) or 10 mg/mL, which can then be diluted to the appropriate working concentrations[1].

Accurate measurement requires the use of proper tools and techniques. For home use, graduated droppers or calibrated syringes provide reasonable accuracy for measuring pre-made solutions. However, it's crucial to verify the starting concentration of your methylene blue source, as products can vary significantly. Professional laboratory settings employ more precise methods, such as UV-Vis spectrophotometry, which measures absorption at 665 nanometers to determine exact concentrations[93].

When preparing or diluting methylene blue solutions, always use distilled water rather than tap water, as minerals and other compounds can interfere with the stability and effectiveness of the solution[1]. For example, to prepare a 0.1 mg/mL solution from a 1 mg/mL stock, mix one part of the stock solution with nine parts of distilled water. This type of dilution requires careful measurement and thorough mixing to ensure uniform distribution.

Proper storage significantly impacts concentration stability. Methylene blue solutions should be kept in amber glass bottles to prevent photo degradation, as exposure to light can alter the concentration and effectiveness over time. Room temperature storage is generally appropriate, but avoid extreme temperatures that could affect stability[1]. Regular visual inspection for any changes in color, clarity, or the presence of particles is essential, as any such changes may indicate degradation and necessitate replacement.

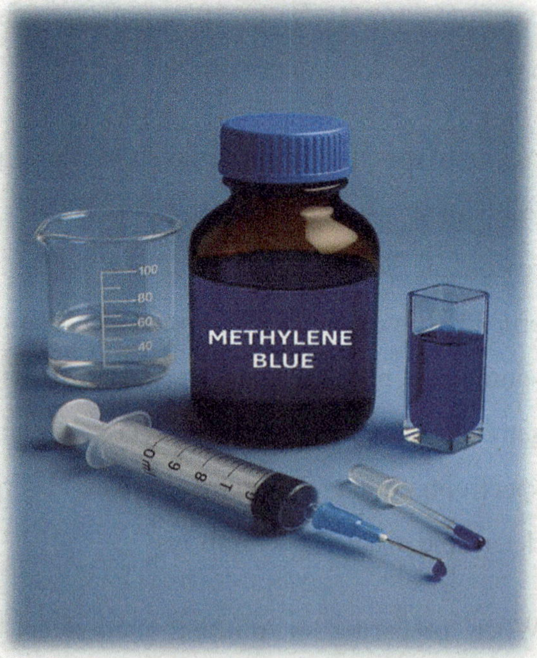

Safety considerations extend beyond accurate measurement. Always wear appropriate protective equipment when handling methylene blue, as it can cause skin and clothing to stain. Label all solutions clearly with concentration, preparation date, and expiration date to prevent dosing errors[1]. Keep detailed records of your measurements and calculations to maintain consistency in your protocol.

The therapeutic window for methylene blue varies depending on the intended use, making accurate concentration crucial. Low-dose protocols typically range from 0.5 to 4.0 mg/kg of body weight, while certain medical procedures may require higher concentrations. However, exceeding recommended concentrations can lead to adverse effects, including increased oxidative stress - the opposite of what we're trying to achieve[95].

When working with methylene blue solutions, be aware that certain substances can interfere with accurate measurement. Strong reducing agents, such as thiosulfate, and certain metals can affect readings and potentially alter the therapeutic effects[94]. If you're using other supplements or medications, maintain appropriate timing intervals to avoid any potential interactions.

For optimal accuracy in measuring methylene blue solutions:

- Use calibrated measuring tools appropriate for your volume needs
- Verify the starting concentration of your methylene blue source
- Document all measurements and calculations
- Store solutions properly to maintain concentration stability
- Check for signs of degradation before each use

Understanding concentration levels and proper measurement forms the foundation of successful methylene blue therapy. By following these guidelines and paying close attention to detail, you can ensure consistent and effective dosing tailored to your specific health goals. Remember that precision in measurement directly correlates with both safety and efficacy. There's no room for guesswork when it comes to therapeutic compounds like methylene blue.

Calculating Individual Dosage Requirements

Determining the right dosage of methylene blue requires careful consideration of multiple factors to ensure both safety and effectiveness. While standardized dosing protocols exist for specific medical conditions, therapeutic supplementation requires a more nuanced approach based on individual characteristics and health goals.

The foundation of accurate methylene blue dosing begins with understanding concentration levels. Most therapeutic-grade methylene blue solutions come in either 1% (10mg/mL) or 0.1% (1mg/mL) concentrations. When calculating your individual dosage, it's essential to verify the concentration of your source solution to avoid dosing errors.

Body weight serves as the primary basis for calculating methylene blue dosage; however, it is essential to use lean body weight rather than total body weight[59]. This distinction is crucial because methylene blue distributes primarily in lean tissue rather than fat stores. For most therapeutic applications, the dosing range is 0.5-4.0 mg per kilogram of lean body weight.

To calculate your lean body weight for proper dosing:

- For men: 50 + 0.9 × (height in cm - 152)
- For women: 45.5 + 0.9 × (height in cm - 152)

Once you've determined your lean body weight, you can calculate your specific dose based on the intended therapeutic application[96 97]. Low-dose protocols typically start at 0.5-1.0 mg/kg for cognitive enhancement and mitochondrial support, while higher doses may be indicated for specific medical conditions under the guidance of a healthcare professional.

Several factors can influence your optimal dosage requirements:

- Kidney and liver function[96 97]
- Age and overall health status
- Concurrent medications
- Specific health conditions
- Time of day and frequency of administration

When beginning methylene blue supplementation, it's prudent to start with the lowest effective dose and gradually increase it as needed, while monitoring your response[98]. This approach, known as dose titration, helps minimize potential side effects while identifying your optimal therapeutic range.

The timing of doses can significantly impact effectiveness. For cognitive enhancement, many practitioners recommend administering supplements in the morning to align with natural circadian rhythms. For other applications, splitting the daily dose into two or three administrations may provide more consistent therapeutic effects[97].

Precise measurement is crucial for accurate dosing. Using calibrated droppers or oral syringes helps ensure consistent administration. For a 1% solution (10mg/mL), each milliliter contains 10mg of methylene blue. Therefore, if your calculated dose is 20mg, you would need 2mL of solution.

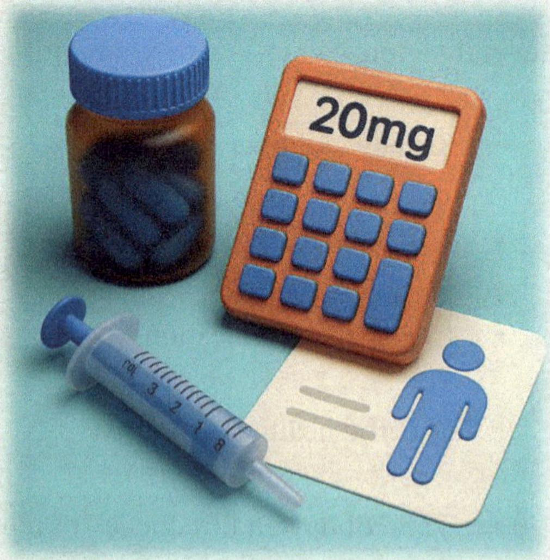

Safety considerations must remain paramount when calculating individual dosage requirements. Never exceed the maximum recommended cumulative dose of 7mg/kg per day, as higher doses may lead to adverse effects. Additionally, certain medical conditions and medications may require dosage adjustments or contraindicate the use of methylene blue entirely[97].

For optimal safety and effectiveness, maintain detailed records of your dosing protocol, including:

- Daily dose amount
- Time of administration
- Effects observed
- Any side effects experienced
- Concurrent supplements or medications

Regular monitoring and assessment of your response to methylene blue helps optimize your individual protocol over time. Pay attention to both immediate effects and long-term changes in your targeted health parameters. This systematic approach allows for evidence-based adjustments to your dosing regimen.

Remember that methylene blue is a potent compound with significant biological effects. While calculating your individual dosage requirements is essential, always consult with a qualified healthcare provider before beginning supplementation, especially if you have underlying health conditions or take prescription medications[96 97 59].

The goal of individualized dosing is to achieve optimal therapeutic benefits while minimizing potential risks. By carefully considering your personal factors, maintaining precise measurements, and following established safety guidelines, you can develop an effective methylene blue protocol tailored to your specific needs.

Timing and Frequency of Administration

The timing and frequency of methylene blue administration play crucial roles in maximizing its therapeutic benefits while minimizing potential risks[95 21 96]. Understanding when and how often to take methylene blue requires careful consideration of several key factors, including your specific health goals, individual response, and overall protocol design.

For cognitive enhancement and general mitochondrial support, morning administration is typically recommended to align with natural circadian rhythms[95]. This timing helps optimize energy production during your most active hours while avoiding potential sleep disruption. The half-life of methylene blue ranges from 5 to 6.5 hours, making morning dosing particularly effective for daytime cognitive benefits.

Frequency of administration varies based on therapeutic goals and dosage levels. For general wellness and cognitive support, once-daily dosing is often sufficient, typically ranging from 0.5 to 2 mg/kg of body weight[96]. Higher therapeutic needs may require divided doses; however, the total daily intake should never exceed 7mg/kg to maintain safety and effectiveness.

Timing considerations should account for potential interactions with other supplements and medications. Methylene blue should be taken on an empty stomach, ideally 30 minutes before or 2 hours after meals to optimize absorption. Additionally, maintain a 4-hour minimum spacing from serotonergic medications or supplements to avoid potential interactions[95 96].

For individuals using methylene blue to treat specific health conditions, the administration timing may need to be more precisely tailored to their individual needs. Therapeutic protocols may require multiple daily doses, typically spaced 4-8 hours apart[99 96], depending on the condition being addressed and individual response patterns. However, such protocols should only be undertaken under the supervision of a professional medical practitioner.

Consider these key timing principles for optimal results:

- Take morning doses within 30 minutes of waking

- Maintain consistent timing daily to establish a routine
- Allow appropriate spacing from meals and other supplements
- Monitor your response to adjust timing as needed
- Document administration times and effects

The frequency of methylene blue administration should be guided by both therapeutic goals and individual response[95]. While some individuals may benefit from daily use, others may achieve optimal results with intermittent administration, such as every other day or several times a week. Regular assessment of your response helps determine the most effective frequency for your needs.

When establishing your methylene blue protocol, start with a conservative approach and gradually adjust based on observed effects[95]. Begin with a single daily dose and monitor your response before considering multiple daily administrations. This methodical approach helps identify your optimal timing while minimizing the risk of adverse effects.

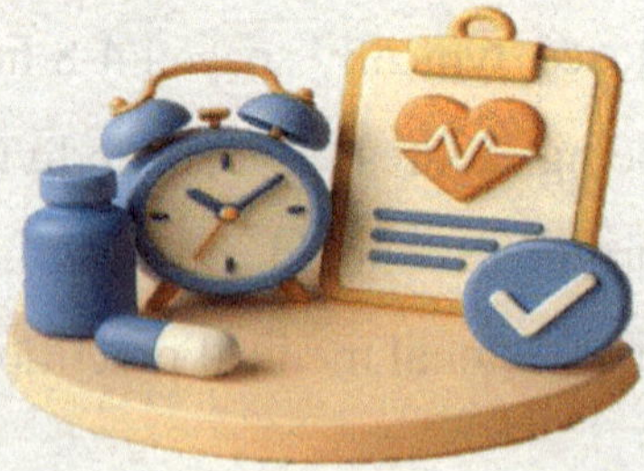

For long-term use, implementing regular "cycling" periods can help maintain effectiveness and prevent potential tolerance development[96]. A common approach is to follow a 5-day-on, 2-day-off schedule, although individual needs may vary. This cycling strategy helps optimize long-term benefits while providing regular assessment periods.

Proper timing also extends to seasonal considerations. Some practitioners recommend adjusting dosing schedules in response to seasonal changes in energy demands and circadian rhythms. For example, earlier morning administration during summer months when days are longer, and slightly later administration during winter months.

Tracking your administration schedule and results is essential for optimizing your protocol. Keep detailed records of:

- Administration times
- Dosage amounts
- Effects observed
- Energy levels throughout the day
- Sleep quality

The success of methylene blue therapy often depends on consistency and precision in timing and frequency[95 96]. While the compound itself is remarkably versatile, its effects can be significantly enhanced through the strategic timing of administration. Regular evaluation and adjustment of your protocol ensures continued effectiveness and optimal results over time.

Remember that individual responses to methylene blue can vary significantly[96]. What works optimally for one person may need adjustment for another. Pay attention to your body's signals and adjust timing and frequency accordingly, always staying within established safety guidelines and consulting with healthcare professionals when needed.

For those new to methylene blue supplementation, these timing guidelines provide a framework for developing an effective protocol. However, remain flexible and willing to adjust based on your experience and specific health goals. The key is finding a sustainable rhythm that maximizes benefits while fitting seamlessly into your daily routine.

Safety Precautions and Contraindications

While methylene blue offers remarkable therapeutic potential, understanding its safety considerations and contraindications is crucial for responsible use[100 102 103]. This powerful compound requires careful attention to proper handling, storage, and administration to minimize risks while maximizing benefits. Whether you're considering methylene blue for cognitive enhancement or other therapeutic purposes, safety must always be your primary consideration.

Methylene blue can interact significantly with certain medications, particularly those affecting serotonin levels in the brain. One of the most critical contraindications is its interaction with selective serotonin reuptake inhibitors (SSRIs), serotonin-norepinephrine reuptake inhibitors (SNRIs), and monoamine oxidase inhibitors (MAOIs). This interaction can potentially lead to serotonin syndrome, a serious condition that requires immediate medical attention[102]. If you're taking any serotonergic medications, it's essential to consult with a healthcare provider before considering methylene blue supplementation.

Certain genetic conditions can also contraindicate the use of methylene blue. Individuals with glucose-6-phosphate dehydrogenase (G6PD) deficiency should avoid methylene blue, as it can trigger hemolytic anemia in this population[102]. This genetic condition affects the stability of red blood cells and requires careful screening before initiating methylene blue therapy.

Proper handling and storage of methylene blue are essential safety considerations. The compound should be stored in tightly closed containers in a cool, dry, well-ventilated area away from direct light exposure[101] [102] [103]. When handling methylene blue, always wear appropriate protective equipment, including gloves and eye protection, as it can cause skin and eye irritation upon direct contact[100 101 103 104].

Dosage precision is critical for safety. While methylene blue has a relatively wide therapeutic window, exceeding recommended doses can lead to adverse effects[100 102]. Start with the lowest effective dose and increase gradually only if needed. Never exceed 7mg/kg per day, as higher doses may increase oxidative stress rather than reduce it.

Special populations require additional precautions. Pregnant and nursing women should avoid methylene blue unless specifically prescribed by a healthcare provider, as its safety during pregnancy and lactation hasn't been fully established. Individuals with severe kidney or liver dysfunction may need dose adjustments or may not be suitable candidates for methylene blue therapy.

Essential safety precautions include:

- Always verify medication interactions before starting methylene blue
- Use pharmaceutical-grade products from reputable sources
- Maintain precise dosing measurements
- Store properly in light-resistant containers

- Keep detailed records of usage and effects

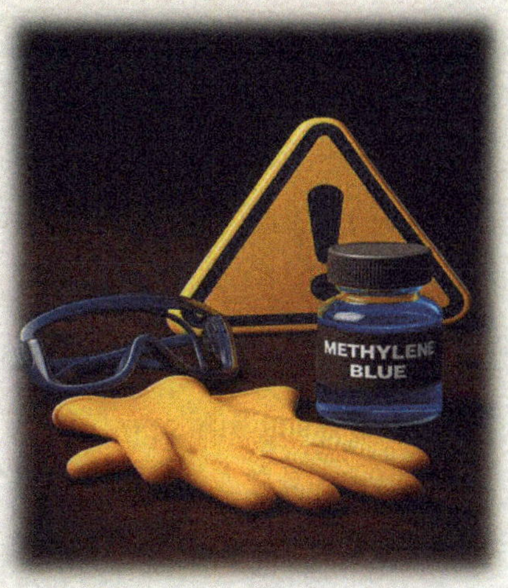

Monitoring for adverse reactions is crucial when using methylene blue. While serious side effects are rare when used appropriately, being aware of potential warning signs helps ensure safe use. Common minor side effects may include temporary discoloration of urine or stool, mild gastrointestinal discomfort, or temporary skin staining[100 103]. However, if you experience symptoms such as confusion, agitation, severe headache, or difficulty breathing, discontinue use immediately and seek medical attention[100 102].

Quality sourcing plays a vital role in safety. Only use pharmaceutical-grade methylene blue from reputable suppliers. Lower-grade products may contain impurities or inconsistent concentrations that could compromise both safety and effectiveness. Always verify the concentration and purity of your methylene blue source before use.

Emergency protocols should be established before administering methylene blue. Keep your healthcare provider's contact information readily available, and ensure that family members or close contacts are aware of your use of methylene blue. In the event of accidental exposure or adverse reactions, having a clear action plan can help prevent complications[100 103 105].

Regular health monitoring is recommended for individuals who use methylene blue on a long-term basis. This may include periodic blood tests to check kidney and liver function, as well as regular assessment of any concurrent medications or supplements. Working with a healthcare provider to establish appropriate monitoring protocols helps ensure continued safe use.

Key contraindications to remember:

- Current use of serotonergic medications[102]
- G6PD deficiency[102]
- Severe kidney or liver dysfunction
- Pregnancy and lactation
- Known hypersensitivity to methylene blue[18]

By following these safety guidelines and understanding contraindications, you can minimize risks while maximizing the therapeutic benefits of methylene blue. Remember that individual responses can vary, and what works safely for one person may not be appropriate for another. Always prioritize safety over convenience, and don't hesitate to consult with healthcare professionals when you have questions about your specific situation.

Drug Interactions and Precautionary Measures

Understanding drug interactions is a critical aspect of safely implementing methylene blue therapy. As a potent monoamine oxidase inhibitor (MAOI), methylene blue can interact significantly with various medications, particularly those that affect serotonin levels in the brain[106 23 109]. These interactions require careful consideration and proper precautionary measures to ensure safe and effective use.

One of the most significant concerns involves the interaction between methylene blue and serotonergic medications. This includes selective serotonin reuptake inhibitors (SSRIs), serotonin-norepinephrine reuptake inhibitors (SNRIs), tricyclic antidepressants (TCAs), and other MAOIs[106 18 23 108 109]. The combination of these medications with methylene blue can potentially lead to serotonin syndrome, a serious and potentially life-threatening condition characterized by agitation, confusion, rapid heartbeat, hypertension, hyperthermia, and muscle rigidity[18 25 109].

The FDA has issued specific guidelines regarding these interactions, recommending that methylene blue should generally be avoided in patients taking serotonergic medications unless required for life-threatening conditions such as methemoglobinemia23. When emergency use is necessary, temporary discontinuation of serotonergic medications may be required under medical supervision[23].

Key medications that interact with methylene blue include:

- SSRIs (fluoxetine, sertraline, citalopram, paroxetine, escitalopram)
- SNRIs (venlafaxine, duloxetine)
- TCAs (amitriptyline, clomipramine)
- MAOIs (phenelzine, selegiline)
- Other antidepressants (bupropion, trazodone, mirtazapine) [106] [18] [23] [108]

Beyond serotonergic medications, methylene blue can also interact with blood pressure medications, potentially reducing the efficacy of nitrates and calcium channel blockers while enhancing the effects of beta-blockers[106]. This interaction requires careful blood pressure monitoring and possible dose adjustments of antihypertensive medications[106].

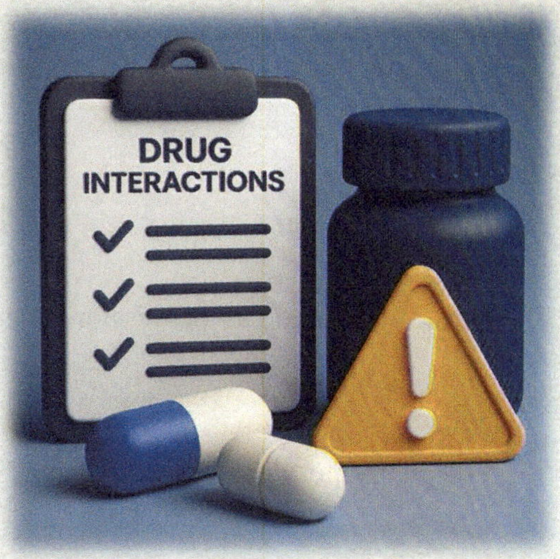

Stimulant medications, including those used for ADHD treatment, may have amplified effects when combined with methylene blue[106]. This can lead to overstimulation, tachycardia, and increased anxiety[106]. Careful monitoring is essential when these combinations cannot be avoided.

Surgical considerations are also important, as methylene blue can interact with various anesthetic agents[106]. Healthcare providers should always be informed about the use of methylene blue before any surgical procedure to prevent potential complications[106].

To ensure safe use of methylene blue, implement these essential precautionary measures:

- Maintain a complete and current medication list[107]
- Consult healthcare providers before starting methylene blue[106 107 18 23]
- Monitor for signs of serotonin syndrome[106 18 25 109]
- Inform all medical professionals involved in your care about methylene blue use
- Follow proper dosing protocols and timing guidelines

Laboratory testing can be affected by the use of methylene blue, making it crucial to inform laboratory staff before any diagnostic tests[110]. The compound can interfere with certain urine and blood tests, potentially leading to inaccurate results.

Special populations require additional precautions. Pregnant and nursing women should avoid methylene blue unless specifically prescribed by a healthcare provider, as safety data in these populations is limited[107 108]. Similarly, individuals with severe kidney or liver dysfunction may require modified protocols or may not be suitable candidates for methylene blue therapy.

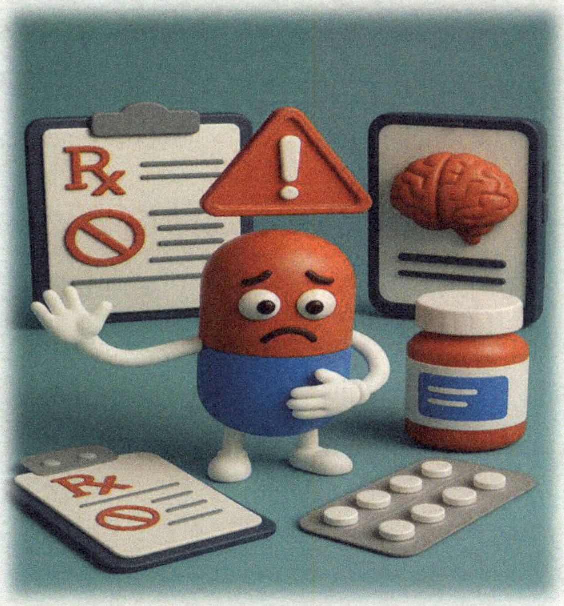

When using methylene blue, maintain vigilant monitoring for any adverse reactions. While serious side effects are rare with appropriate use, being aware of warning signs helps ensure safety. Common minor effects may include temporary urine discoloration or mild gastrointestinal discomfort. However, if you experience confusion, severe headache, difficulty breathing, or other concerning symptoms, discontinue use immediately and seek medical attention.

Quality sourcing plays a crucial role in minimizing interaction risks. Use only pharmaceutical-grade methylene blue from reputable suppliers, as lower-grade products may contain impurities or inconsistent concentrations that could compromise both safety and effectiveness.

Establish clear emergency protocols before beginning methylene blue use. Keep healthcare provider contact information readily available, and ensure that family members or close contacts are aware of your use of methylene blue. Having a clear action plan can help prevent complications in the event of adverse reactions.

For long-term users, regular health monitoring is recommended, including periodic assessment of kidney and liver function, particularly when using other medications concurrently. Working with healthcare providers to establish appropriate monitoring protocols helps ensure the continued safe use of medications while minimizing the risk of adverse interactions.

Proper Storage Conditions and Shelf Life

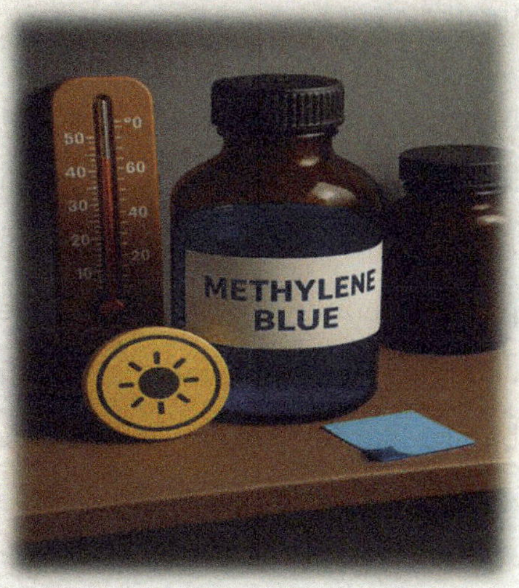

Proper storage of methylene blue is crucial for maintaining its therapeutic potency and ensuring safety over time. The compound's remarkable stability, when stored correctly, allows for an indefinite shelf life - but only under specific environmental conditions that protect its chemical integrity and effectiveness[112].

Temperature control plays a crucial role in maintaining the stability of methylene blue. The compound should be stored in cool, dry conditions, away from extreme heat sources that could trigger decomposition[112]. While methylene blue demonstrates impressive thermal stability up to its melting point of 190°C, routine storage should maintain much lower temperatures to prevent degradation of the compound's therapeutic properties[100].

Light exposure represents another critical factor affecting the long-term stability of methylene blue. The compound should be stored in amber glass bottles or other light-resistant containers to prevent photo degradation. This protection from light helps maintain the compound's chemical structure and ensures consistent therapeutic effects over time[112].

Moisture control is crucial for maintaining the integrity of methylene blue. Storage containers must remain tightly sealed to prevent humidity from compromising the compound's stability[112]. For crystalline or powder forms, any visible changes in physical appearance, such as clumping or color changes from the characteristic dark green with a bronze-like luster, may indicate moisture contamination and potential degradation[112].

When storing prepared solutions, additional considerations come into play. While pure methylene blue powder demonstrates indefinite stability, aqueous solutions require more careful monitoring. Solutions should be prepared using distilled water rather than tap water to prevent potential chemical interactions that could affect stability. Commercial preparations typically carry a 36-month shelf life recommendation, although this often represents a conservative estimate rather than the actual degradation timeline[111].

Proper storage location is equally important for maintaining the stability of methylene blue. The storage area should be:

- Well-ventilated to prevent dust accumulation
- Separated from incompatible materials

- Protected from direct sunlight
- Away from food and beverages
- Secured from unauthorized access

Container selection has a significant impact on long-term stability. Glass containers are preferred over plastic, as they offer better protection against environmental factors and prevent potential chemical interactions. Containers should be thoroughly cleaned and dried before use. Any transfer of methylene blue between containers should occur in a clean, controlled environment[112].

Regular quality assessment of stored methylene blue is recommended. Visual inspection can reveal potential degradation signs, including:

- Changes in color intensity
- Formation of precipitates
- Unusual odors
- Moisture presence
- Container damage or deterioration

Proper labeling is essential for safe storage management. Each container should clearly indicate:

- Concentration and form
- Preparation date (for solutions)
- Expiration date (if applicable)
- Storage requirements
- Safety precautions

Environmental monitoring of storage conditions helps ensure optimal preservation of the product. Temperature and humidity logs can track storage conditions over time, particularly in professional or clinical settings where maintaining precise environmental parameters is crucial[100].

Safety considerations during storage extend beyond maintaining chemical stability. Proper ventilation prevents dust accumulation that could create explosion risks in powder forms[100]. Additionally, storage areas should include appropriate safety equipment and protective gear for handling, such as gloves and eye protection[112].

For long-term storage management, implement these key practices:

- Regular inventory checks
- Rotation of stock based on preparation dates

- Documentation of environmental conditions
- Periodic quality assessments
- Proper disposal of expired materials

When storing multiple forms or concentrations of methylene blue, maintain clear separation and labeling to prevent confusion or mixing. Different forms may have varying stability profiles and storage requirements, making proper organization essential for safety and effectiveness[111].

Proper disposal of expired or compromised methylene blue requires professional waste management services[100]. Never dispose of the compound or its containers with regular household waste, as this could pose environmental and safety risks. Maintain relationships with licensed waste disposal services for proper handling of any materials requiring disposal[100].

By following these storage guidelines and maintaining proper environmental conditions, you can ensure the continued stability and effectiveness of your methylene blue supply. Regular monitoring and documentation of storage conditions help prevent degradation while maintaining safety and therapeutic potency over time.

Quality Assessment and Degradation Signs

Quality assessment of methylene blue is fundamental to ensuring both safety and therapeutic effectiveness[116]. Understanding how to evaluate the quality of your methylene blue and recognizing signs of degradation helps maintain optimal benefits while preventing potential risks associated with a compromised product.

The purity and stability of methylene blue can be assessed through several key indicators. High-quality methylene blue should maintain its characteristic deep blue color without fading or discoloration. Any shift toward a brownish tint or significant color variation may indicate oxidation or photo degradation. Similarly, the solution should remain clear without precipitation or cloudiness, as these changes can signal chemical breakdown or contamination.

Chemical stability is crucial for the therapeutic effectiveness of a compound. Pharmaceutical-grade methylene blue undergoes rigorous testing using advanced analytical techniques like high-performance liquid chromatography coupled with tandem mass spectrometry (LC-MS/MS). This method can detect even trace amounts of impurities or degradation products[115], ensuring the highest quality standards. While such sophisticated testing isn't available to most users, understanding basic quality indicators helps maintain product integrity.

Proper quality assessment begins with sourcing. Obtain methylene blue only from reputable suppliers that provide certificates of analysis and adhere to Good Manufacturing Practices (GMP). These certifications help ensure consistent purity and potency. When receiving new Methylene Blue, carefully inspect the product and documentation before use.

Key physical indicators of quality degradation include:

- Changes in color intensity or hue
- Formation of precipitates or cloudiness
- Unusual odors
- Visible contamination
- Changes in solution viscosity

Maintaining quality requires proper storage conditions. Methylene blue should be kept in amber glass bottles or other light-resistant containers to prevent photo degradation. The storage area should maintain a consistent room temperature (20-25°C) and remain dry to prevent moisture-induced degradation. Proper sealing of containers helps minimize exposure to air and potential oxidation.

Regular quality assessment should become part of your methylene blue protocol. Before each use, visually inspect the solution for any changes in appearance, clarity, or color. If stored as a powder, check for any clumping or color changes from the characteristic dark green with bronze-like luster. Any significant changes should be carefully evaluated before use.

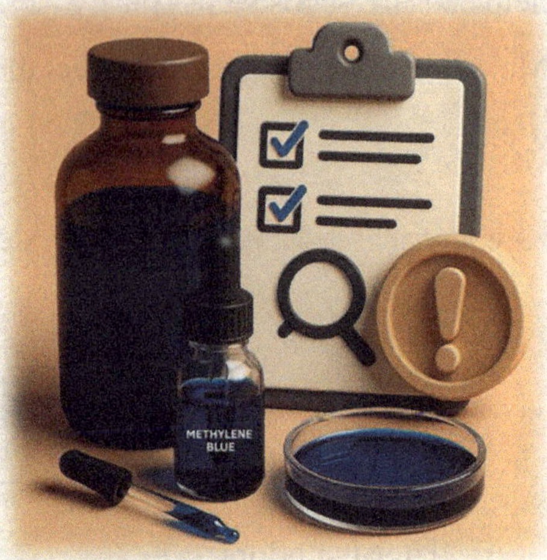

The shelf life of properly stored methylene blue can be quite extensive, but this depends heavily on storage conditions and form. While pure methylene blue powder demonstrates remarkable stability, solutions typically carry more conservative expiration recommendations. Commercial preparations typically have a 36-month shelf life, although this may be extended under optimal storage conditions.

Quality monitoring should include regular documentation of:

- Visual inspection results
- Storage conditions
- Date of receipt or preparation

- Any observed changes
- Batch numbers and supplier information

When evaluating the quality of methylene blue, consider both physical and chemical indicators. While advanced analytical testing may not be readily available, careful attention to basic quality parameters helps maintain product integrity. Never use methylene blue that shows signs of degradation, as a compromised product may not only be less effective but could also pose safety risks.

Spectrophotometric methods offer an additional tool for quality assessment, particularly in laboratory or clinical settings. These techniques can measure precise concentrations and detect potential impurities, with detection limits as low as 0.02 mg/L[113 114]. While such testing may not be practical for individual users, understanding these quality control measures helps appreciate the importance of proper handling and storage.

Maintaining methylene blue quality requires a systematic approach to storage and handling. Implement these essential practices:

•Store in appropriate containers away from light

•Maintain consistent temperature conditions

- Minimize air exposure

- Keep detailed records
- Regularly inspect for quality changes

By understanding and monitoring these quality indicators, you can ensure the continued effectiveness of your methylene blue protocol while maintaining safety standards[115 116]. Remember that quality assessment is not a one-time event, but an ongoing process that requires regular attention and documentation.

Emergency Protocol and First Aid Measures

Understanding and implementing proper emergency protocols for methylene blue is crucial for ensuring safety during therapeutic use. While methylene blue demonstrates an excellent safety profile when used correctly, having clear emergency procedures and first aid measures in place helps prevent complications. It ensures a prompt and appropriate response to any adverse events that may occur.

Exposure to methylene blue can happen through various routes, each requiring specific first aid measures. Inhalation of methylene blue powder or concentrated solutions can irritate the respiratory tract. If inhalation occurs, immediately move to fresh air. If breathing becomes difficult, seek emergency medical attention. Artificial respiration or oxygen may be required in severe cases[117 100 119].

Skin contact with methylene blue typically causes temporary staining but can also result in mild irritation. If skin exposure occurs, thoroughly rinse the affected area with copious amounts of water for 15-20 minutes. Remove any contaminated clothing and wash it separately before reuse[117 100]. While skin staining may persist for several days, it is generally harmless and will fade naturally over time.

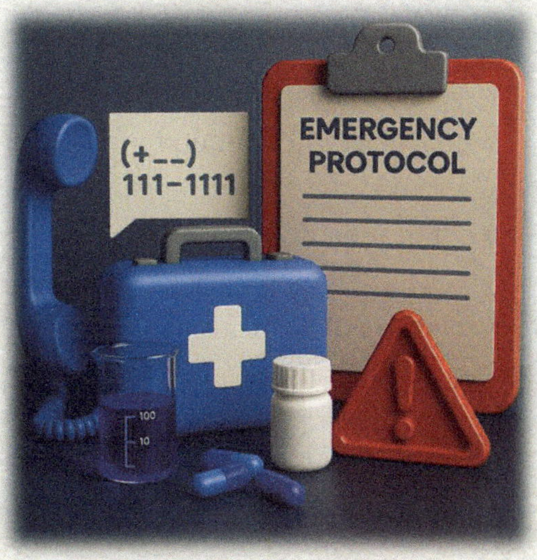

Eye exposure requires immediate attention as methylene blue can cause significant irritation to ocular tissues. If eye contact occurs, flush your eyes thoroughly with water for at least 10-15 minutes while keeping your eyelids open. If contact lenses are present, remove them if they can be done easily[117 100]. Continue rinsing and seek medical attention if irritation persists.

Accidental ingestion of methylene blue solutions requires careful management and attention. If ingestion occurs, rinse mouth thoroughly with water. Do not induce vomiting unless directed explicitly by medical professionals. Drink plenty of water to aid dilution. Monitor for symptoms such as nausea, vomiting, or abdominal pain[117 119]. Seek immediate medical attention if large quantities are ingested or if symptoms become severe.

Essential emergency protocols should include:

- Immediate discontinuation of methylene blue use
- Documentation of exposure circumstances
- Recording of any symptoms experienced
- Contact information for emergency services
- Location of nearest emergency medical facility

Proper preparation can significantly improve emergency response outcomes. Maintain a well-stocked first aid kit that includes:

- Clean water for rinsing
- Sterile eye wash solution
- Protective gloves
- Clean towels or cloths
- Emergency contact information

Recognizing signs of adverse reactions is crucial for proper emergency response. While serious reactions are rare with therapeutic doses, certain symptoms warrant immediate medical attention:

- Severe headache or confusion
- Difficulty breathing
- Rapid heart rate
- High blood pressure
- Muscle rigidity
- Severe agitation

Particularly concerning is the potential for serotonin syndrome when methylene blue is combined with serotonergic medications. This serious condition requires immediate medical intervention[118]. Symptoms may include:

- Mental status changes
- Neuromuscular abnormalities
- Autonomic hyperactivity
- Hyperthermia

- Seizures

For healthcare settings, additional emergency protocols should be established:

- Clear documentation procedures
- Emergency response team notification protocols
- Equipment and medication accessibility
- Staff training requirements
- Patient monitoring guidelines

Prevention remains the best emergency protocol. Maintain detailed records of methylene blue use, including:

- Dosage amounts and timing
- Batch numbers and sources
- Any concurrent medications
- Previous reactions or sensitivities
- Regular health monitoring results

Emergency protocols should be regularly reviewed and updated to ensure their continued effectiveness. Staff training and emergency response drills help maintain readiness for potential adverse events[102]. Regular assessment of emergency equipment and supplies ensures availability when needed.

In the event of exposure or adverse reactions, having clear communication protocols is crucial. Ensure all relevant parties know:

- Who to contact in emergencies
- What information to provide
- Where to access medical care
- How to document incidents
- When to escalate response measures

Proper storage and handling procedures help prevent emergencies before they occur. Always maintain methylene blue in appropriate containers, clearly labeled with safety information and emergency protocols[102]. Keep safety data sheets readily available for reference in the event of an emergency.

By implementing these comprehensive emergency protocols and first aid measures, users of methylene blue can ensure proper response to potential adverse events while maintaining the safety and effectiveness of their therapeutic protocols. Regular review and updates of these procedures help maintain preparedness and optimize emergency response outcomes.

Record Keeping and Dose Tracking Methods

Maintaining detailed records of methylene blue administration is crucial for ensuring both safety and optimal therapeutic outcomes[96 95]. Proper documentation enables precise dosing, helps identify patterns in effectiveness, and provides crucial information for healthcare providers. This systematic approach to tracking becomes especially vital when implementing long-term methylene blue protocols or adjusting doses based on individual response.

Accurate record keeping begins with documenting essential data points for each administration. These include the exact dose (in mg or mg/kg), form of administration (solution, tablet, or other), concentration of the preparation, and precise timing of each dose[96 95 121]. Additionally, tracking physiological responses, any side effects, and concurrent medications[95] helps build a comprehensive picture of individual response patterns and potential interactions.

Implementing a structured tracking system requires choosing appropriate tools and methods. Digital platforms offer convenience and automated features[120 95], while traditional paper logs provide reliability and simplicity[96 95]. Many practitioners recommend maintaining both digital and physical records to ensure redundancy and accessibility.

Essential elements to track in your methylene blue protocol include:

- Exact dose amounts and timing[96 95 121]
- Form and concentration used[96 95 121]
- Route of administration[96 122]
- Batch or lot numbers
- Physiological responses[95]
- Any side effects observed[95]
- Concurrent medications[96]
- Overall effectiveness

Digital tracking methods have revolutionized the management of

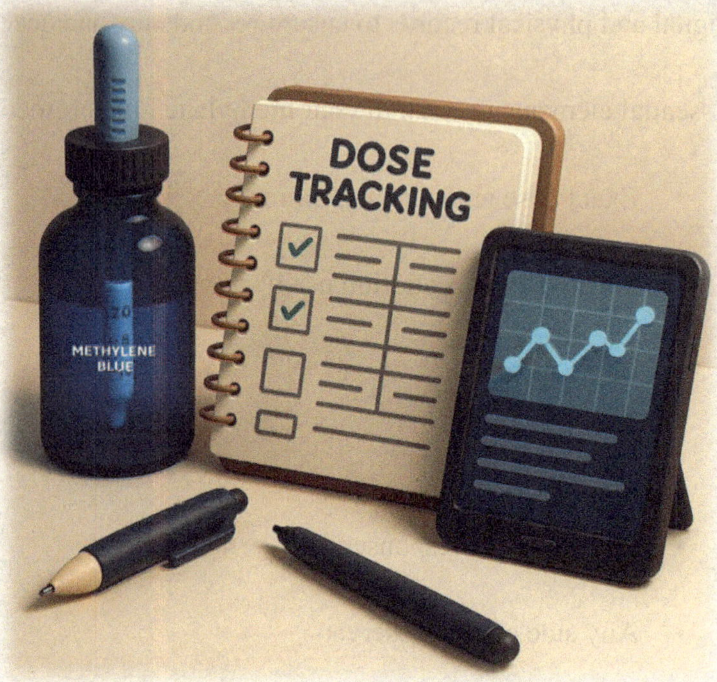

methylene blue protocols. Electronic medical records and specialized apps can automatically calculate doses, flag potential interactions, and generate trend analyses[120 95]. These tools often include built-in safety features that warn of dosing errors or dangerous drug combinations, adding an extra layer of protection to your protocol.

For home use, maintaining a comprehensive but straightforward tracking system proves invaluable. Whether using a dedicated notebook, spreadsheet, or mobile app, consistency in recording is key. Document each dose immediately after administration to ensure accuracy and completeness of records.

Physiological monitoring becomes particularly important when adjusting methylene blue protocols. Regular tracking of vital signs, cognitive effects, and energy levels helps optimize dosing schedules and amounts[95]. This data provides concrete evidence of effectiveness and helps identify any necessary adjustments to the protocol.

When documenting side effects or unusual responses, include specific details about timing, severity, and duration[95]. This information proves crucial for healthcare providers in assessing the appropriateness of current protocols and making necessary adjustments. Even minor effects should be noted, as patterns may emerge over time that inform optimal dosing strategies.

For clinical settings, standardized documentation protocols ensure consistency across different administrators and shifts. These typically include:

- Patient identifiers and relevant health conditions[96]
- Precise dosing calculations and verifications[96 95 121]
- Administration times and routes[96 122]
- Monitoring parameters and results[95]
- Administrator identification

- Any adverse events or reactions[95]

Regular review of accumulated data helps identify trends and optimize protocols over time[120 95]. Monthly or quarterly assessments can reveal patterns in effectiveness, timing of peak benefits, or subtle side effects that might otherwise go unnoticed. This systematic analysis supports evidence-based adjustments to maximize therapeutic benefits while maintaining safety.

Quality control measures should be integrated into any tracking system to ensure accuracy and reliability. Regular verification of recorded data, backup procedures for digital records, and periodic review of documentation completeness help maintain the integrity of your tracking system. This attention to detail supports both safety and optimization of methylene blue protocols.

When tracking multiple aspects of methylene blue use, consider organizing data into distinct categories:

- Dosing records
- Physiological responses
- Side effect monitoring
- Effectiveness measures

- Protocol adjustments

Proper record keeping extends beyond individual dose tracking to include storage conditions, product quality assessments, and supply management. Maintaining records of purchase dates, lot numbers, and storage conditions helps ensure product integrity and supports proper rotation of stock.

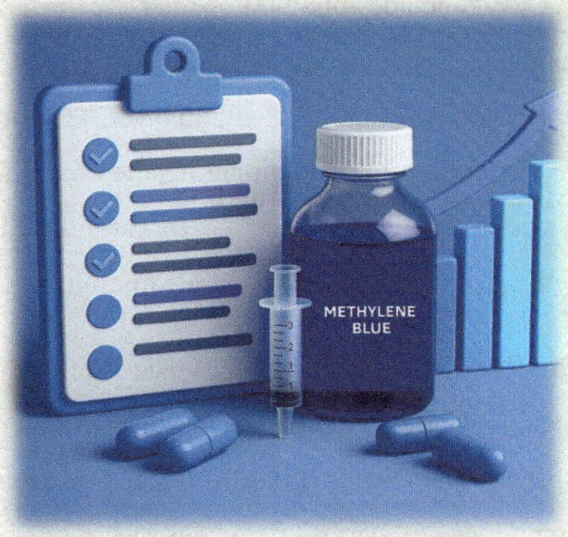

For research or clinical applications, additional documentation requirements may apply[96] [95]. These often include more detailed monitoring parameters, standardized assessment tools, and specific reporting protocols. Always verify applicable requirements for your particular setting or application.

By implementing comprehensive record-keeping and dose-tracking methods, you establish a solid foundation for the safe and effective use of methylene blue. This systematic approach not only enhances safety but also supports optimal therapeutic outcomes through careful monitoring and evidence-based protocol adjustments.

As we conclude this vital chapter on the practical implementation of methylene blue therapy, it's essential to reflect on the critical protocols and safety measures we've explored. The journey from understanding proper dosing to maintaining detailed records forms the foundation of successful methylene blue use. By carefully adhering to these guidelines, you can maximize benefits while minimizing potential risks.

Proper dosing remains the cornerstone of methylene blue therapy. We've examined how individual factors such as body weight, health status, and specific therapeutic goals influence optimal dosing strategies. The importance of starting with conservative doses and gradually adjusting based on individual response cannot be overstated. Remember that precision in measurement and consistency in timing play crucial roles in achieving desired outcomes.

Safety considerations extend beyond just proper dosing. We've explored critical drug interactions, particularly with serotonergic medications, and emphasized the importance of consulting healthcare providers before beginning methylene blue supplementation. Understanding storage requirements, quality assessment methods, and proper handling techniques ensures both safety and therapeutic effectiveness.

Proper storage and handling of methylene blue solutions deserve special attention. Temperature control, protection from light exposure, and the selection of an appropriate container all contribute to maintaining the compound's stability and effectiveness. Regular quality assessments help identify any signs of degradation before they can impact therapeutic outcomes.

Emergency protocols and first aid measures provide an essential safety net for individuals using methylene blue. While serious adverse reactions are rare with proper use, having clear response procedures in place ensures immediate and appropriate action if needed. The documentation we've discussed supports both safety and optimization of therapeutic protocols.

Detailed record keeping emerges as a crucial component of successful methylene blue therapy. Tracking doses, responses, and any side effects creates a valuable dataset for optimizing individual protocols. This systematic approach to documentation supports both safety and effectiveness while providing essential information for healthcare providers.

As you begin implementing methylene blue therapy, precision matters. Success depends on accurate dosing, proper storage, and consistent documentation—all essential for achieving reliable, safe results.

Regularly reviewing and adjusting your protocol in response to individual feedback ensures continued effectiveness over time.

The framework outlined in this chapter provides clear, evidence-based guidance for using methylene blue safely and effectively. By applying these principles with attention to your unique physiology and health goals, you can fully leverage its therapeutic potential.

Methylene blue therapy is inherently individualized. Stay disciplined with dosing and monitoring, adhere to safety protocols, and collaborate with qualified healthcare professionals to refine your approach as needed.

In the next chapter, we'll explore how to amplify methylene blue's benefits through strategic lifestyle integration, combining it with nutrition, exercise, and complementary wellness practices to maximize results while maintaining the safety standards established here.

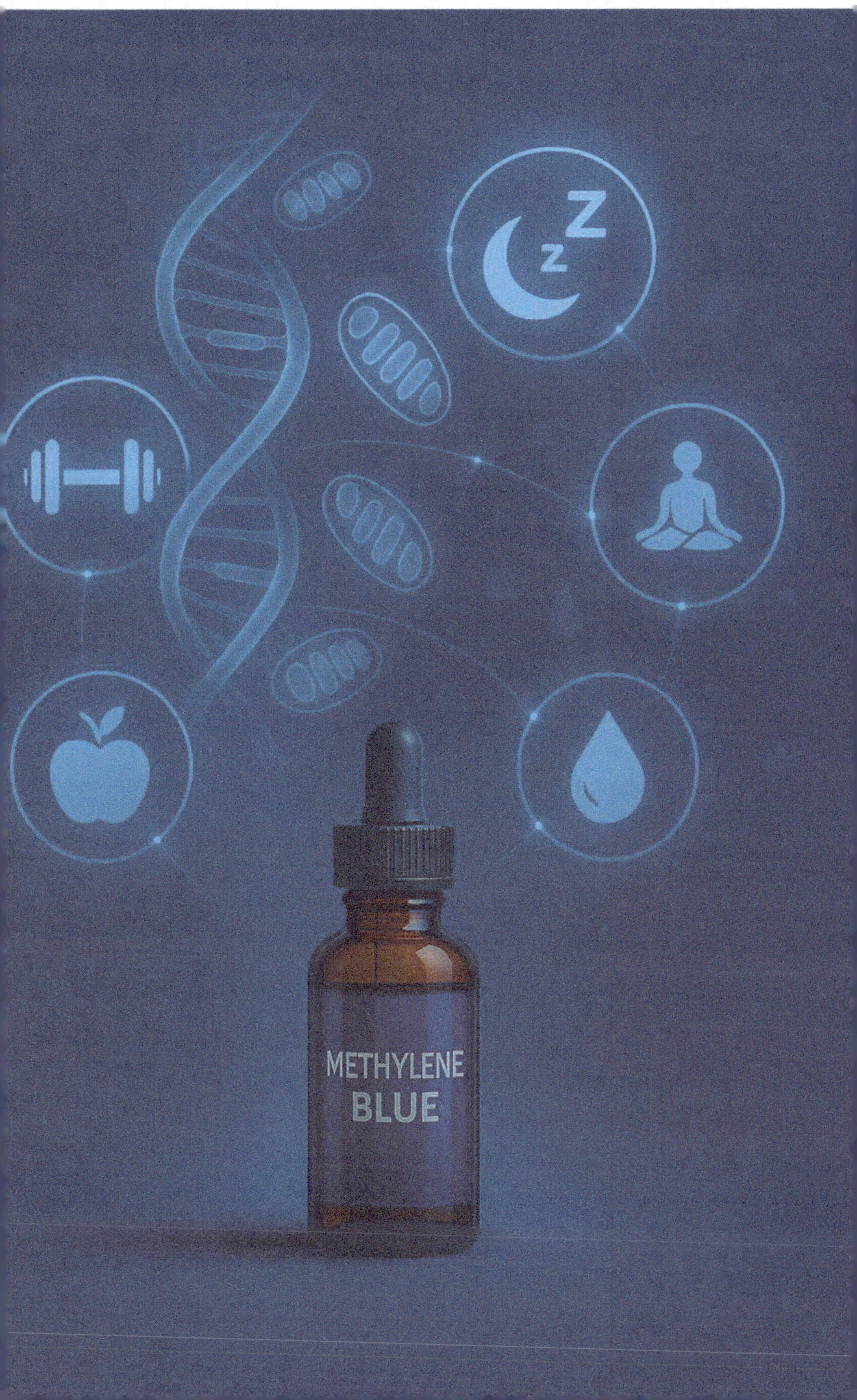
METHYLENE
BLUE

CHAPTER 5

OPTIMIZING YOUR RESULTS: COMBINING METHYLENE BLUE WITH LIFESTYLE STRATEGIES

The true potential of methylene blue emerges when it's integrated into a broader health and wellness strategy. Like a conductor leading an orchestra, its timing and coordination with lifestyle practices can produce a powerful symphony of benefits. This compound doesn't work in isolation; its therapeutic power is amplified through synergy with exercise, nutrition, sleep, and stress management.

Biological synchronicity is key. When supplementation aligns with the body's natural rhythms and supportive habits, methylene blue's cellular-enhancing effects reach their full potential.

In this chapter, we'll outline the essential components of a holistic optimization strategy, from exercise timing and nutritional pairing to restorative sleep and stress resilience. Each factor contributes to a framework that maximizes methylene blue's benefits. You'll see how lifestyle choices can either enhance or blunt its effects, and how to tailor a protocol that fits your personal goals.

This isn't just about timing; it's about creating an integrated system that sustains cellular health and energy production. Whether your focus is cognitive enhancement, mitochondrial support, or general vitality, the principles here will help you build a more effective, sustainable regimen.

As we move forward, we'll translate the science into practical steps: coordinating methylene blue with exercise for peak performance, pairing it with nutrient-rich foods for better absorption, and syncing supplementation with your body's rhythms for maximum impact.

Exercise Timing and Performance Enhancement

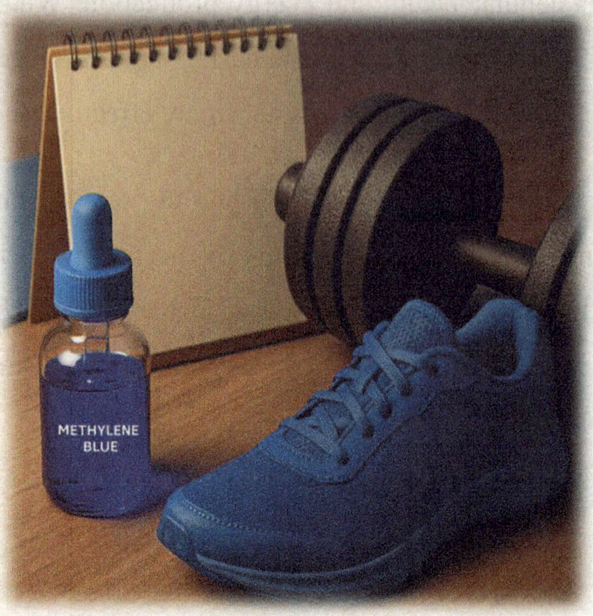

The strategic timing of methylene blue consumption in relation to exercise can significantly enhance athletic performance and recovery[123 124 78 53]. When properly coordinated, methylene blue's ability to optimize mitochondrial function and improve oxygen utilization creates a powerful foundation for enhanced physical performance[123 124 78]. Understanding the science behind this synergy allows us to maximize the benefits while maintaining safety and effectiveness.

At its core, methylene blue works by enhancing the electron transport chain within our mitochondria, the cellular powerhouses responsible for producing ATP energy[123 125]. When taken 30-60 minutes before exercise, methylene blue can increase ATP production efficiency, providing more readily available energy for muscular contractions and sustained activity[123 124 78]. This timing allows the compound to reach peak blood levels just as physical activity begins, optimizing its performance-enhancing effects.

The dosing strategy for exercise enhancement typically starts at 0.5-2 mg per kilogram of body weight[123], though it's essential to begin at the lower end of this range and gradually adjust based on individual response[123 124]. Morning workouts tend to be ideal for methylene blue supplementation, as this timing aligns with our natural circadian rhythms and helps avoid any potential sleep disruption that could occur with evening use[124].

Methylene blue's impact on oxygen utilization represents another crucial mechanism for exercise enhancement. By improving how efficiently our cells use oxygen during physical exertion, we can help delay the onset of fatigue and extend the time before reaching the lactate threshold[124 78]. This benefit is particularly valuable for endurance activities where maintaining aerobic metabolism is crucial for sustained performance[78].

The compound's antioxidant properties also play a crucial role in enhancing exercise performance and promoting recovery. During intense physical activity, our bodies generate increased oxidative stress and accumulate lactic acid. Methylene blue helps buffer these effects, potentially reducing muscle soreness and supporting faster recovery between training sessions[123 78 53]. However, it's crucial to note that individuals taking serotonergic medications should avoid methylene blue due to the risk of serious interactions[124].

Optimal results are achieved by combining methylene blue supplementation with a balanced diet and adequate hydration. Foods that support mitochondrial health, such as avocados, eggs, fatty fish, and dark leafy greens, can enhance the compound's effectiveness[124]. Adequate hydration becomes especially important when using methylene blue, as it can influence oxygen handling and blood volume dynamics during exercise[124].

For athletes considering methylene blue supplementation, it's worth noting that while the compound is not currently listed on the World Anti-Doping Agency's banned substance list, it's essential to verify its status with the specific sport's governing bodies[78]. Additionally, those using other performance supplements should carefully evaluate potential interactions and adjust their timing accordingly[124 78].

A practical protocol for exercise enhancement with methylene blue includes:

- Take 0.5-2 mg/kg body weight 30-60 minutes before exercise[123 124 78]

- Start with the lowest effective dose and adjust as needed[123 124]
- Prioritize morning workouts for optimal timing[124]
- Maintain proper hydration before, during, and after exercise[124]
- Support with mitochondrial-friendly nutrition[124]
- Monitor individual response and adjust protocol as needed[124 78]

The key to success lies in consistency and careful attention to timing. While methylene blue can significantly enhance exercise performance[123 124 78 53], it's most effective when integrated into a comprehensive approach to training and recovery. Regular monitoring of response and adjusting protocols based on individual needs ensures optimal results while maintaining safety and effectiveness.

Nutritional Synergies and Optimal Combinations

The effectiveness of methylene blue can be significantly enhanced through strategic nutritional combinations and timing. Understanding these synergistic relationships allows for optimized therapeutic outcomes while supporting the compound's primary mechanisms of action within cellular systems. By carefully selecting complementary nutrients and dietary approaches, we can create an environment that maximizes the benefits of methylene blue.

One of the most powerful nutritional synergies exists between methylene blue and vitamin C. When these compounds interact within the body, they form leukomethylene blue. This enhanced antioxidant compound delivers superior protective effects compared to either substance alone[128]. This biochemical transformation enhances the ability of both substances to neutralize free radicals, thereby creating a more robust defense mechanism against cellular oxidative stress[128].

The practical implications of this combination extend beyond simple antioxidant protection. The enhanced free radical scavenging activity provides comprehensive protection for mitochondria, the cellular powerhouses that methylene blue specifically targets[128]. However, it's crucial to approach this combination with careful consideration of dosing, as high amounts of either compound could potentially lead to unintended physiological effects[128].

Intermittent fasting represents another powerful synergistic approach when combined with methylene blue supplementation. Both interventions impact mitochondrial function and cellular stress resistance pathways, creating a complementary effect that enhances overall health outcomes[127]. While methylene blue directly improves mitochondrial efficiency, intermittent fasting triggers metabolic switching and cellular mechanisms that promote resilience against stress[127]

Supporting methylene blue's function with NAD+ precursors provides another layer of cellular optimization. NAD+ serves as an essential coenzyme that fuels cellular repair and optimizes energy levels, working in conjunction with

methylene blue's electron transport enhancement properties[129]. This combination creates a comprehensive approach to energy production and cellular rejuvenation[129].

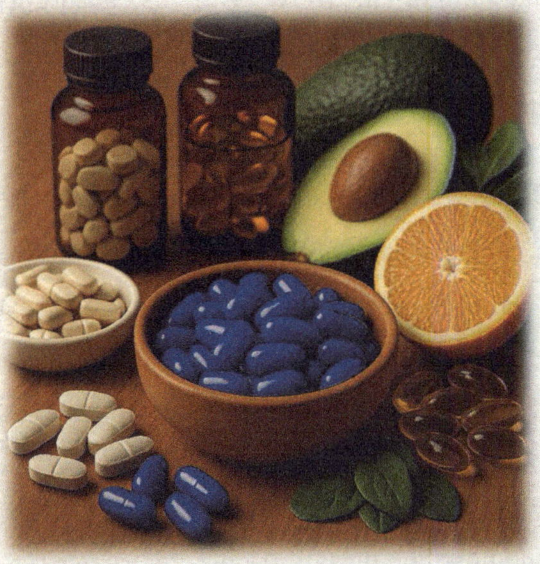

Key nutritional combinations that support methylene blue include:

- Vitamin C for enhanced antioxidant effects
- CoQ10 for additional mitochondrial support

- B-vitamins for optimal energy metabolism
- Omega-3 fatty acids for cellular membrane health
- Magnesium for enhanced ATP production

The timing of nutrient combinations plays a crucial role in maximizing benefits. For optimal absorption and effectiveness, methylene blue should typically be taken on an empty stomach, separated from foods or supplements that might interfere with its absorption. However, supporting nutrients can be strategically timed throughout the day to maintain cellular support.

Antioxidant defense systems become particularly important when using methylene blue, as the compound's ability to decrease reactive oxygen species (ROS) can be enhanced through comprehensive antioxidant support[126]. This creates a multi-layered approach to protecting cells from oxidative damage while supporting mitochondrial biogenesis[126].

When implementing nutritional synergies with methylene blue, several key principles should guide the approach:

- Start with basic combinations before adding complexity
- Monitor individual response to different combinations
- Maintain consistent timing of supplementation

- Ensure adequate hydration throughout the day
- Consider the circadian rhythm when timing doses

Safety considerations remain paramount when combining methylene blue with other nutrients[128]. Individuals taking serotonergic medications should exercise particular caution and seek professional guidance before implementing any combination protocol. Additionally, individuals with specific health conditions or those taking other medications should consult their healthcare providers to ensure safe implementation.

The integration of methylene blue with proper nutrition creates a foundation for optimal cellular health[126]. By understanding and implementing these synergistic relationships, we can enhance the compound's therapeutic potential while supporting overall health outcomes. Remember that individual responses may vary, and a personalized approach often yields the best results.

Practical Protocol Summary:

- Begin with methylene blue alone to establish a baseline response
- Gradually introduce the vitamin C combination
- Implement supporting nutrients based on individual needs
- Time doses around meals and other supplements

- Monitor and adjust based on personal response

By thoughtfully combining methylene blue with complementary nutrients and dietary strategies, we create an environment that allows cellular health to truly flourish[126]. This integrated approach supports not just the immediate effects of methylene blue but also its long-term benefits for overall health and vitality.

Sleep Optimization Strategies

The relationship between methylene blue and sleep optimization represents a crucial intersection in maximizing the compound's therapeutic potential. While methylene blue is primarily known for its cognitive-enhancing and mitochondrial-supporting properties, understanding its interaction with sleep patterns and circadian rhythms can significantly impact overall treatment outcomes. When properly timed and combined with evidence-based sleep strategies, methylene blue can support both daytime performance and nighttime recovery[130 19].

The timing of methylene blue administration plays a crucial role in optimizing sleep. Unlike traditional stimulants that can disrupt sleep architecture, low-dose methylene blue taken early in the day supports cognitive function without compromising sleep quality[130]. This unique characteristic stems from its mechanism of action, which enhances mitochondrial efficiency rather than directly manipulating neurotransmitter systems[130].

Mitochondrial health and circadian regulation share an intimate connection that influences sleep quality. By supporting mitochondrial efficiency, methylene blue may contribute to improved energy metabolism during waking hours and more restorative sleep at night[130 19]. This biological synchronization becomes particularly important when developing a comprehensive sleep optimization strategy.

Implementing evidence-based sleep optimization strategies alongside methylene blue usage can enhance overall outcomes. Key components include:

- Maintaining a consistent sleep-wake schedule to reinforce circadian rhythms
- Managing light exposure with morning sunlight and evening blue light reduction
- Optimizing sleep environment through temperature, darkness, and noise control
- Implementing mindful nutrition and hydration practices
- Incorporating stress reduction and relaxation techniques[130 19]

The practical implementation of sleep optimization while using methylene blue requires careful attention to timing and individual response. Morning administration of methylene blue, typically between

6:00 AM and 10:00 AM, enables optimal cognitive enhancement during daytime hours while supporting natural sleep-wake cycles[130]. This timing aligns with our natural circadian rhythms, helping to prevent potential sleep disruptions.

Nutritional considerations also play a crucial role in optimizing sleep when using methylene blue. Supporting cellular energy systems through proper nutrition can enhance both the compound's effectiveness and sleep quality. Key nutritional strategies include maintaining adequate

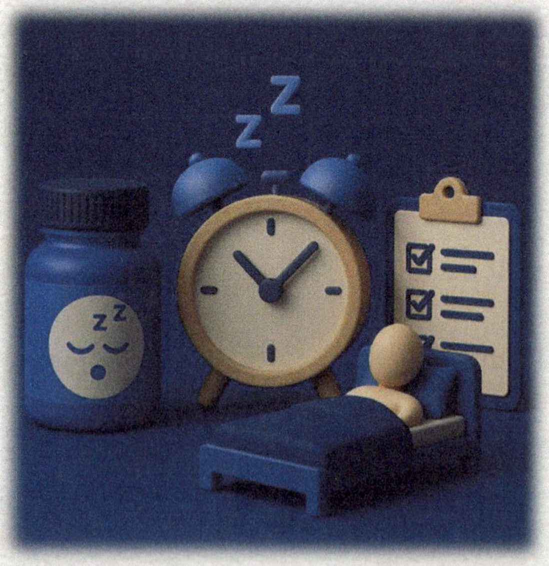

hydration, ensuring sufficient mineral intake, particularly magnesium and timing larger meals away from bedtime.

Physical activity represents another crucial component of sleep optimization for individuals using methylene blue. Regular exercise, particularly when completed several hours before bedtime, promotes deeper sleep and enhances mitochondrial function[19]. This complementary effect can amplify the cellular benefits of methylene blue while supporting overall sleep architecture.

A comprehensive protocol for sleep optimization while using methylene blue includes:

- Morning administration of methylene blue (ideally before 10:00 AM)[130]
- Exposure to natural light within 30 minutes of waking
- Regular physical activity, completed 3-4 hours before bedtime[19]
- Consistent sleep and wake times, even on weekends
- Creation of a cool, dark, quiet sleep environment

Monitoring individual response becomes essential when implementing these strategies. While most users report no sleep disruption with morning methylene blue administration, individual variability exists[130]. Tracking sleep quality through objective measures (such as sleep duration and nighttime awakenings) and subjective measures (such as morning alertness and daytime energy levels) can help optimize personal protocols.

The synergistic relationship between methylene blue and sleep extends beyond simple rest and recovery. By supporting mitochondrial function during the day, methylene blue may enhance the efficiency of nighttime cellular repair processes[130] [19]. This optimization of cellular energy systems can create a positive feedback loop, where better sleep supports enhanced daytime function, and improved daytime metabolism supports more restorative sleep.

Safety considerations remain paramount when implementing sleep optimization strategies with methylene blue. Individuals with pre-existing sleep disorders or those taking medications that affect sleep should consult healthcare providers before combining interventions. Additionally, those sensitive to stimulants may need to adjust timing or dosage to prevent any impact on sleep quality.

By understanding and implementing these sleep optimization strategies, methylene blue users can maximize the benefits of the compound while supporting overall health and recovery. The key lies in creating a structured approach that respects individual variation while maintaining consistency in core sleep-supporting practices. This balanced methodology ensures optimal outcomes while minimizing potential disruptions to natural sleep patterns.

Stress Management and Mindfulness Integration

The intersection of methylene blue supplementation with stress management and mindfulness practices represents a powerful approach to optimizing both mental and physical well-being[131 132 84]. While methylene blue works at the cellular level to enhance mitochondrial function and reduce oxidative stress[131 132 133], mindfulness practices provide complementary benefits that can amplify these effects. Understanding this synergistic relationship enables us to develop more effective protocols for managing stress while promoting overall brain health.

Methylene blue's biochemical effects on stress reduction operate through several key mechanisms. As a potent antioxidant, it helps neutralize the free radicals that accumulate during periods of chronic stress[131 133 27]. This protection is particularly important in the brain, where oxidative damage can impair cognitive function and emotional regulation[27 134]. Additionally, methylene blue's ability to enhance mitochondrial efficiency helps maintain cellular energy production during stressful periods when metabolic demands are high[131 132 133].

The compound's neuroprotective properties complement mindfulness practices by creating a more resilient neurobiological environment. Research indicates that methylene blue can help stabilize mood and reduce anxiety without the risk of dependency or significant side effects[85 132 84]. This makes it an excellent partner for mindfulness-based interventions, as both approaches work to enhance emotional regulation and stress resilience through different but complementary pathways[132 84 134].

Integrating mindfulness practices with methylene blue supplementation requires careful attention to timing and dosage. Morning administration of methylene blue, typically between 0.5-2mg per kilogram of body weight, provides cognitive support throughout the day while allowing for natural wind-down in the evening[85]. This timing aligns well with traditional mindfulness practices, which often emphasize morning meditation or breathing exercises.

Key mindfulness practices that synergize with methylene blue include:

- Focused breathing exercises for stress reduction
- Body scan meditation for physical tension release
- Mindful movement practices like gentle yoga
- Present-moment awareness training
- Stress-response monitoring techniques

The biochemical support provided by methylene blue can enhance the effectiveness of these mindfulness practices by optimizing brain function and energy metabolism[131 133 27]. When cells have adequate energy and protection from oxidative stress, the brain is better equipped to maintain focus and emotional balance during mindfulness exercises[133 134].

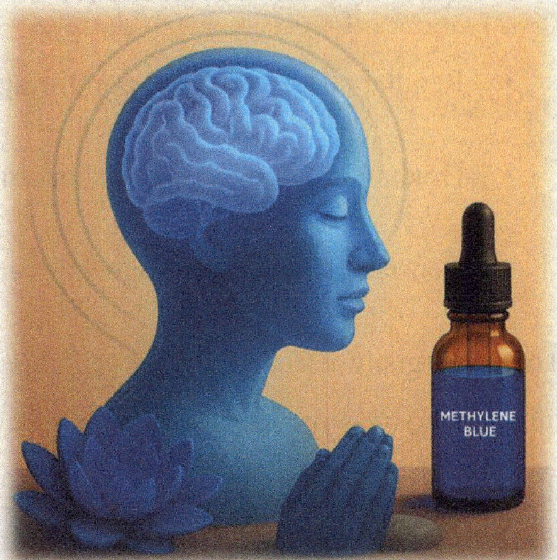

Safety considerations remain paramount when combining methylene blue with stress management practices. Individuals taking serotonergic medications, including many common antidepressants, should avoid methylene blue due to potential interactions[132 84]. Additionally, those with anxiety disorders should start with lower doses and gradually increase based on individual response.

A comprehensive protocol for integrating methylene blue with stress management includes:

- Morning methylene blue administration (0.5-2mg/kg)[85]

- Daily mindfulness practice (15-30 minutes)
- Regular stress response monitoring
- Gradual protocol adjustment based on results
- Consistent sleep-wake schedule maintenance

The synergistic effects of this combined approach extend beyond immediate stress reduction. By supporting both cellular resilience and psychological adaptation, this integration creates a foundation for long-term stress management and improved mental health outcomes[132 84 134]. The antioxidant and neuroprotective properties of methylene blue help maintain cognitive clarity during mindfulness practices[131 133 27], while the calming effects of mindfulness support optimal cellular function[134].

Monitoring progress becomes essential when implementing this combined approach. Key indicators of success include:

- Reduced perceived stress levels
- Improved emotional regulation
- Enhanced cognitive clarity
- Better stress recovery time
- Increased mindfulness capacity

Practical implementation strategies should focus on consistency and gradual progression. Beginning with lower doses of methylene blue and shorter mindfulness sessions allows for proper assessment of individual response[85]. As tolerance and comfort develop, both aspects can be adjusted to optimize benefits while maintaining safety.

The integration of methylene blue with mindfulness practices represents a powerful approach to stress management that addresses both the biological and psychological aspects of stress resilience[132 84 134]. By combining the cellular-protective effects of methylene blue with the cognitive-behavioral benefits of mindfulness, individuals can develop more robust stress management capabilities, thereby supporting long-term brain health[131 132 133 27].

Circadian Rhythm Alignment

The intricate dance between our body's internal clock and environmental rhythms plays a crucial role in optimizing health outcomes, particularly when using therapeutic compounds like methylene blue. Understanding and aligning these biological rhythms can significantly enhance the effectiveness of methylene blue while supporting overall well-being. The timing of methylene blue administration becomes especially important when considering its effects on cellular energy production and cognitive function.

Methylene blue's interaction with circadian rhythms operates through several key mechanisms. By enhancing mitochondrial function in retinal cells improves the capacity to receive and transmit light signals to the brain, which are essential for maintaining proper circadian alignment[135]. This enhancement of cellular energy systems creates a foundation for more robust circadian signaling throughout the body.

The relationship between methylene blue and light exposure represents a critical consideration for optimal timing. Morning administration of methylene blue, particularly when combined with natural sunlight exposure, can help reinforce healthy circadian patterns[135]. This timing aligns with the body's natural tendency toward heightened alertness and metabolic activity during daylight hours.

Key strategies for optimizing circadian rhythm with methylene blue include:

- Morning administration (ideally before 10:00 AM)
- Intentional exposure to natural sunlight during supplementation
- Reduction of artificial blue light exposure in evening hours[137 140]
- Maintenance of consistent sleep-wake cycles
- Strategic timing of exercise and meals

The pineal gland plays a central role in circadian regulation through its production of melatonin[135 138]. Methylene blue's antioxidant properties may help protect the pineal gland from calcification and oxidative stress, supporting its ability to maintain proper circadian signaling[135]. This protection becomes particularly important in our modern environment, where various factors can disrupt natural circadian patterns.

Molecular research suggests that methylation processes are crucial for maintaining circadian rhythm stability[136]. While methylene blue's effects on methylation are complex, its support of mitochondrial function and cellular energy production provides a foundation for maintaining stable circadian patterns. This cellular support becomes especially important when considering the metabolic demands of maintaining proper circadian alignment.

Practical implementation requires careful attention to timing and environmental factors. A comprehensive protocol should include:

- Consistent morning methylene blue administration
- Regular exposure to natural light, especially at sunrise[135]
- Minimization of artificial light exposure after sunset[137]
- Support for pineal gland health through complementary strategies[135]

- Regular monitoring of sleep quality and energy patterns

Safety considerations remain paramount when implementing circadian optimization strategies with methylene blue. Individuals taking medications that affect sleep or circadian rhythms should consult healthcare providers before combining interventions. Additionally, individuals sensitive to stimulants may need to adjust their timing to prevent disruption to their natural sleep patterns.

The synergistic effects of proper circadian alignment and methylene blue extend beyond immediate benefits. By supporting both cellular energy production and natural biological rhythms, this approach establishes a foundation for enhanced cognitive function, improved metabolic health, and overall vitality[135] [139]. The key lies in maintaining consistency while respecting individual variation in response.

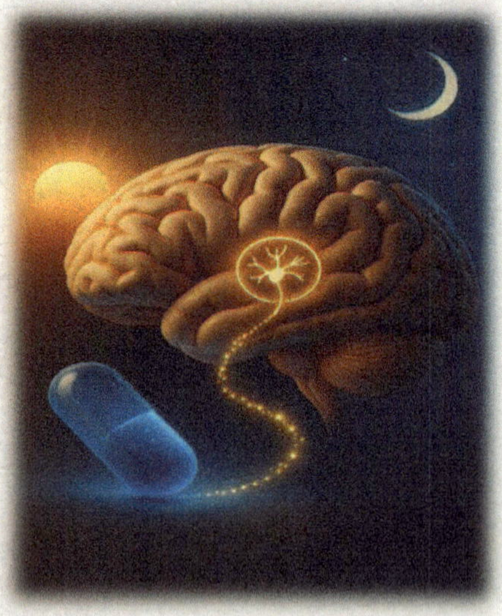

Metabolic health particularly benefits from proper circadian alignment when using methylene blue. Research indicates that circadian disruption can impair glucose metabolism and reduce insulin sensitivity[137]. By supporting proper timing of methylene blue administration and maintaining consistent circadian patterns, these metabolic processes can be optimized.

Protocol Summary:

- Administer methylene blue in the morning (0.5-2mg/kg)
- Ensure exposure to natural light within 30 minutes of waking[135]
- Maintain consistent meal and exercise timing
- Create a dark, cool environment for sleep
- Monitor individual response and adjust timing as needed

By understanding and implementing these circadian alignment strategies, methylene blue users can maximize the compound's benefits while supporting overall health and vitality. The key lies in creating a structured approach that respects both biological rhythms and individual variation while maintaining consistency in core practices. This balanced methodology ensures optimal outcomes while minimizing potential disruptions to natural circadian patterns.

Hydration and Detoxification Support

The relationship between methylene blue therapy and proper hydration represents a critical foundation for optimizing therapeutic outcomes. Methylene blue's effectiveness relies heavily on adequate fluid levels for optimal distribution throughout the body's tissues and efficient elimination of metabolic byproducts. Understanding this relationship allows us to maximize benefits while supporting the body's natural detoxification processes.

Methylene blue requires sufficient fluid volume for proper cellular distribution, particularly given its unique ability to cross the blood-brain barrier and accumulate in mitochondria[144]. Water serves as the primary medium for transporting methylene blue to target tissues, especially the brain, where it can enhance oxygen consumption by 35-70%[141 142]. This increased metabolic activity generates additional demands on the body's fluid balance, making proper hydration essential for both the delivery of nutrients and the removal of waste.

The compound's interaction with cellular detoxification systems represents a sophisticated relationship that requires careful consideration. As a powerful antioxidant, methylene blue helps neutralize free radicals and reduce oxidative stress while supporting the body's natural detoxification processes[141 143]. This antioxidant capacity becomes particularly important as cellular energy production increases, generating more metabolic byproducts that require efficient elimination.

The liver plays a central role in processing methylene blue and managing its therapeutic effects. As the primary organ for drug metabolism, the liver converts methylene blue into various metabolites that require proper hydration for efficient elimination. Supporting liver function through adequate fluid intake becomes essential for optimal results, particularly when using methylene blue for extended periods.

Key hydration strategies for methylene blue therapy include:

- Consistent water intake throughout the day
- Monitoring urine color and output[141]
- Maintaining electrolyte balance
- Supporting kidney function
- Avoiding dehydrating substances

The dramatic increase in mitochondrial activity induced by methylene blue results in a corresponding increase in cellular waste products. By enhancing the electron transport chain and promoting mitochondrial function[141], methylene blue increases metabolic activity, which must be supported through proper hydration. This enhanced cellular respiration generates byproducts requiring efficient clearance through multiple elimination pathways.

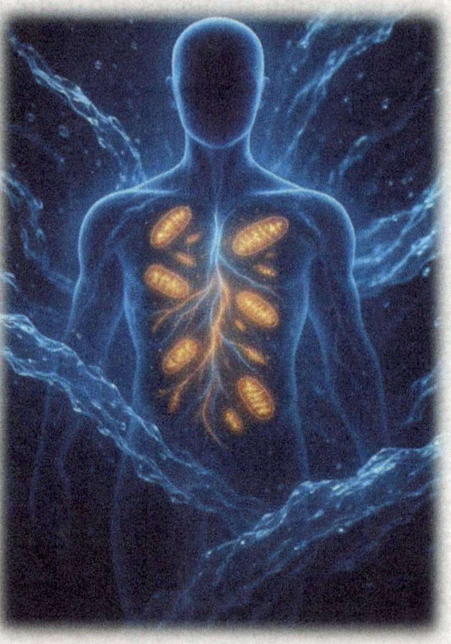

Methylene blue's ability to increase NAD+ production[142] further amplifies cellular energy production and metabolic activity. This increased activity, while beneficial, requires robust hydration support to facilitate the transport and elimination of metabolic waste products. Adequate fluid intake ensures that these enhanced metabolic processes can operate efficiently without creating unnecessary stress on elimination organs.

The timing of hydration becomes particularly important when implementing methylene blue therapy. Pre-treatment hydration ensures adequate fluid volume for distribution, while ongoing hydration supports elimination processes and may help minimize potential side effects such as nausea or headaches[141]. The characteristic blue-tinted urine that occurs with methylene blue use provides a visible marker for monitoring both compound elimination and hydration status[141].

Supporting natural elimination pathways requires attention to multiple bodily systems. The kidneys represent the primary route of elimination for methylene blue metabolites, while the lymphatic system helps manage cellular debris and inflammatory byproducts[143]. Both systems require proper hydration to function optimally and maintain efficient waste removal.

Practical Protocol for Hydration Support:

- Begin with 8-10 glasses of filtered water daily
- Increase intake based on activity and climate
- Monitor urine color and frequency[141]
- Support electrolyte balance
- Maintain a consistent daily hydration schedule

Safety considerations remain paramount when implementing hydration protocols with methylene blue. Individuals taking serotonergic medications should avoid methylene blue entirely[141], regardless of hydration status. Individuals with kidney or liver conditions should consult their healthcare providers before starting therapy, as these organs play a crucial role in processing and eliminating the compound.

The integration of proper hydration with methylene blue therapy creates a foundation for optimal outcomes. By supporting both delivery and elimination processes, adequate hydration helps maximize therapeutic benefits while minimizing potential side effects. Regular monitoring and adjustment of hydration protocols based on individual response ensures sustained effectiveness over time.

Long-term success with methylene blue therapy relies on establishing sustainable hydration practices. Rather than implementing intensive short-term interventions, developing consistent daily habits that support fluid balance and elimination pathways provides more reliable results. This approach particularly benefits those using methylene blue for anti-aging or cognitive enhancement purposes[142 143], where sustained therapy may be desired.

By understanding and implementing these hydration and detoxification support strategies, methylene blue users can optimize their therapeutic outcomes while maintaining safety and effectiveness. The key lies in creating a structured approach that respects individual variation while maintaining consistency in core hydration practices. This balanced methodology ensures optimal results while supporting the body's natural detoxification processes.

Supplement Stacking Guidelines

The strategic combination of methylene blue with other supplements requires careful consideration of safety, timing, and potential interactions[145 63]. Understanding these relationships allows for optimized therapeutic outcomes while maintaining safety and effectiveness. When properly implemented, supplement stacking can enhance the benefits of methylene blue while supporting overall health and cellular function.

The foundation of successful supplement stacking with methylene blue begins with the principle of "start low and go slow." Initial doses should range from 0.5 to 1 mg when introducing new supplement combinations to assess individual tolerance[145 122]. This cautious approach allows for careful monitoring of effects while minimizing the risk of adverse reactions.

Certain combinations require special attention due to their potential for hazardous interactions. Methylene blue should never be combined with serotonergic medications, including SSRIs, MAOIs, or serotonin-boosting herbs, due to the risk of potentially life-threatening serotonin syndrome[145 147]. This extends to supplements that significantly impact neurotransmitter systems, particularly those affecting dopamine or norepinephrine levels[124 147].

Optimal absorption and effectiveness require strategic timing of methylene blue administration. The compound should be taken on an empty stomach, either 30 minutes before or two hours after meals[122]. This timing consideration extends to other supplements in the stack, as certain combinations may either enhance or interfere with absorption.

Synergistic supplement combinations that can safely enhance methylene blue's benefits include:

- Coenzyme Q10 (CoQ10) for enhanced mitochondrial support[145] [148]
- NAD+ precursors to boost cellular energy production[145] [126]
- B-vitamins for mitochondrial enzyme support[124] [148]
- Omega-3 fatty acids for brain health[148]
- Glutathione and other antioxidants for enhanced cellular protection[124] [148] [126]

The implementation of supplement stacking requires careful attention to hydration status. Adequate fluid intake becomes particularly important when combining supplements, as dehydration can exacerbate potential side effects like headache or nausea[122] [124]. Regular monitoring of hydration status through urine color and output provides valuable feedback for adjusting the protocol.

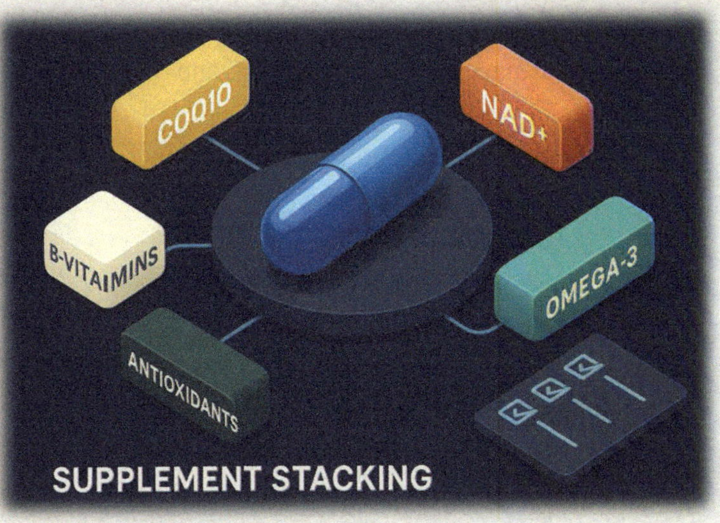

Cycling supplement combinations help prevent the development of tolerance while maintaining effectiveness. A typical approach involves using methylene blue and its complementary supplements for 1-3 months, followed by a rest period of 1-2 months[146]. This cycling strategy helps optimize benefits while reducing the risk of side effects or diminished response.

Practical implementation requires systematic monitoring and documentation. Maintaining a daily journal of doses, timing, effects, and any side effects helps identify optimal protocols while ensuring safety[122].

This documentation becomes particularly valuable when adjusting combinations or introducing new supplements to the stack.

Key considerations for successful supplement stacking include:

- Use only pharmaceutical-grade methylene blue[122]
- Maintain consistent timing of administration[122]
- Monitor individual response to combinations
- Ensure adequate hydration throughout the day[122 124]
- Document effects and adjust protocols as needed[122]

Nutritional support plays a crucial role in optimizing supplement stacks with methylene blue. Foods rich in healthy fats, antioxidants, and micronutrients can enhance the effectiveness of supplement combinations while supporting overall cellular health[124]. This nutritional foundation becomes particularly important when implementing more complex stacking protocols.

Safety remains paramount when combining supplements with methylene blue. Beyond avoiding serotonergic agents, caution should be exercised with other strong nootropics or stimulants due to the risk of overstimulation and unpredictable interactions[124 145]. Individual tolerance should be well-established before attempting more complex combinations.

A basic protocol for implementing supplement stacks includes:

- Morning administration of methylene blue (0.5-1 mg initially)[145][122]
- Strategic timing of complementary supplements
- Consistent hydration throughout the day[122][124]
- Regular monitoring of response and side effects[122]
- Periodic assessment of protocol effectiveness

By understanding and implementing these supplement stacking guidelines, methylene blue users can optimize their therapeutic outcomes while maintaining safety and effectiveness. The key lies in creating a structured approach that respects individual variation while maintaining consistency in core practices. This balanced methodology ensures optimal results while minimizing potential risks associated with supplement combinations.

Environmental Factors and Exposure Optimization

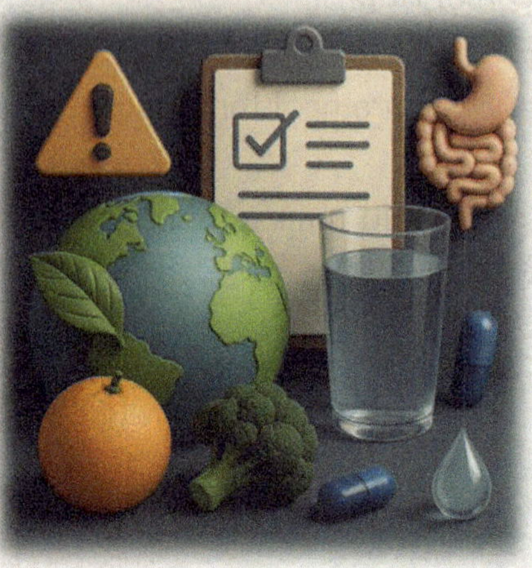

The effectiveness of methylene blue therapy can be significantly influenced by various environmental factors that affect its absorption, metabolism, and overall therapeutic potential. Understanding and optimizing these environmental conditions creates a foundation for maximizing benefits while minimizing potential complications. From pH levels to pollutant exposure, each factor plays a crucial role in how methylene blue interacts with cellular systems.

The chemical environment, particularly pH and salinity levels, has a profound impact on the stability and bioavailability of methylene blue. Research has demonstrated that optimal conditions for methylene blue transformation occur at specific pH levels, with studies showing peak activity at pH 3.6[11 49]. While these findings stem from environmental research, they underscore the importance of maintaining a proper pH balance through dietary and lifestyle choices when using methylene blue therapeutically.

Pollutant exposure represents another critical factor in optimizing the use of methylene blue. The compound's complex structure and interaction with other environmental toxins necessitate careful attention to reducing overall toxic burden[150]. This becomes particularly important in regions with poor water quality or high industrial pollution, where environmental exposure to synthetic dyes and other pollutants may impact the therapeutic efficacy of methylene blue.

Key environmental factors affecting methylene blue include:

- pH and electrolyte balance
- Exposure to environmental pollutants
- Microbiome composition and health
- Hydration status
- Overall toxic burden

The gut microbiome plays a surprisingly important role in methylene blue metabolism. Research has shown that certain microorganisms can transform methylene blue[149], potentially affecting its bioavailability and therapeutic effects. This understanding highlights the importance of maintaining a healthy gut environment through proper nutrition and probiotic support when using methylene blue therapeutically.

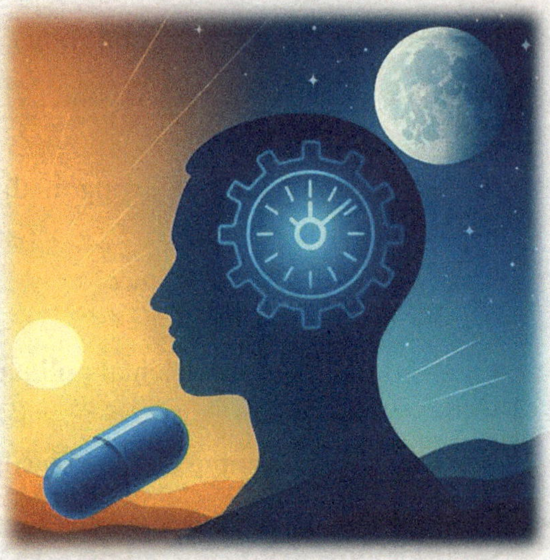

Optimizing environmental conditions for methylene blue therapy requires a multi-faceted approach. Maintaining adequate hydration becomes particularly important, as water serves as both a medium for methylene blue distribution and a crucial component of its elimination. Proper hydration supports the renal excretion of methylene blue and its metabolites while helping to maintain an optimal electrolyte balance[149].

Dietary considerations play a vital role in environmental optimization. A diet rich in antioxidants and low in processed foods can help mitigate oxidative stress, potentially widening the therapeutic window of methylene blue. Additionally, avoiding concurrent exposure to other synthetic dyes or environmental toxins through careful food and water choices supports optimal outcomes[150].

Practical strategies for environmental optimization include:

- Regular monitoring of hydration status
- Consumption of filtered water to reduce toxin exposure
- Implementation of detoxification support practices
- Maintenance of healthy gut flora through diet and probiotics
- Reduction of exposure to environmental pollutants

The relationship between environmental factors and the efficacy of methylene blue extends to cellular detoxification systems. Supporting the body's natural detoxification pathways through lifestyle practices that enhance liver and kidney function becomes crucial for optimal results. This includes regular exercise, moderate alcohol intake, and avoidance of hepatotoxic substances.

Safety considerations remain paramount when implementing environmental optimization strategies. Individuals living in areas with poor water quality or high industrial pollution may need to take additional precautions to minimize exposure to environmental toxins that could interact with methylene blue[150]. Regular monitoring of responses and adjustments to protocols based on individual environmental conditions ensures optimal outcomes.

A comprehensive protocol for environmental optimization includes:

- Daily consumption of filtered water
- Regular support of detoxification pathways
- Maintenance of proper electrolyte balance
- Reduction of exposure to synthetic dyes and pollutants
- Support of a healthy gut microbiome

By understanding and implementing these environmental optimization strategies, methylene blue users can enhance therapeutic outcomes while maintaining safety and effectiveness. The key lies in creating a structured approach that addresses multiple environmental factors while maintaining consistency in core practices. This balanced methodology ensures optimal results while supporting the body's natural regulatory systems.

Long-term success with methylene blue therapy relies on sustained attention to environmental factors. Rather than implementing intensive short-term interventions, developing consistent daily habits that support optimal environmental conditions provides more reliable results. This approach is particularly beneficial for individuals using methylene blue for ongoing health optimization or therapeutic purposes, where sustained effectiveness is crucial.

Creating Your Personalized Protocol

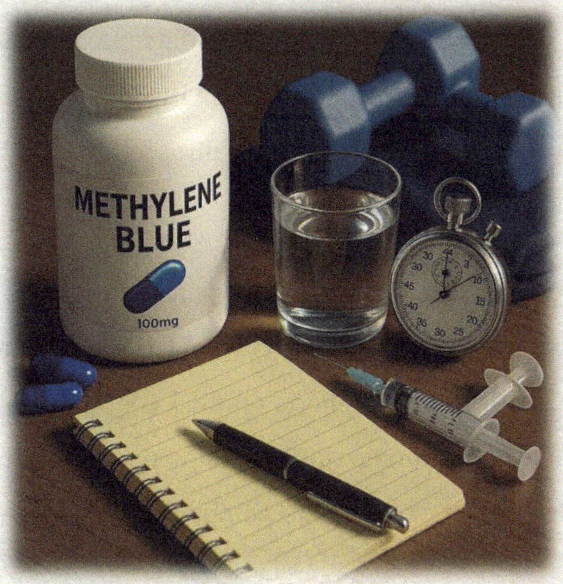

Creating an effective personalized protocol for methylene blue requires careful consideration of multiple factors, including dosage, timing, and individual health status. The key to success lies in developing a systematic approach that accounts for your specific needs while adhering to established safety guidelines. By understanding the fundamental principles of methylene blue administration and combining them with appropriate lifestyle strategies, you can optimize its therapeutic potential.

The foundation of any personalized protocol begins with proper dosing. Research indicates that therapeutic doses typically range from 1 to 2 mg/kg of body weight, with specific applications requiring different concentrations[95 121]. For acquired methemoglobinemia, the standard dose is 1 mg/kg administered intravenously over 5 to 30 minutes[95 121]. For vasoplegic syndrome, a dose of 2 mg/kg infused over 20 minutes is recommended[95].

Timing plays a crucial role in the development of protocols. Morning administration, typically between 6:00 AM and 10:00 AM, aligns with natural circadian rhythms and supports optimal cognitive enhancement throughout the day. This timing strategy helps prevent potential sleep disruption while maximizing the compound's energy-enhancing properties.

Essential components of a personalized protocol include:

- Precise dosage calculation based on body weight
- Strategic timing of administration
- Adequate hydration support
- Regular monitoring of the response

- Documentation of effects and adjustments

Safety considerations must remain paramount when developing your protocol. Individuals taking serotonergic medications, including SSRIs and MAOIs, should avoid methylene blue entirely due to the risk of serious interactions[121]. Those with G6PD deficiency must also abstain from use, as it can trigger hemolytic anemia[121] [68]. Pregnant and breastfeeding women should exercise particular caution and consult healthcare providers before implementation[121].

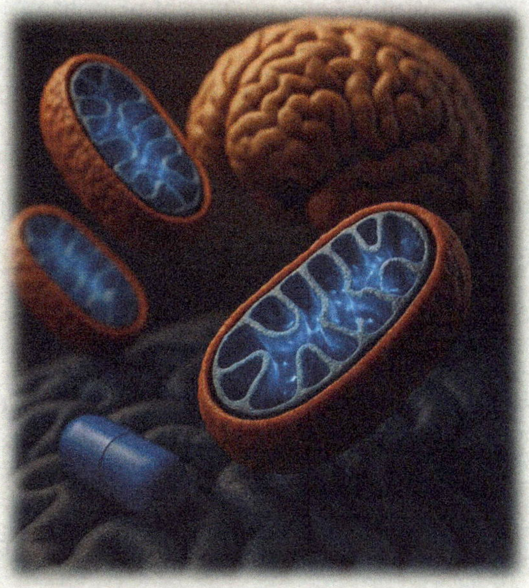

The integration of lifestyle strategies enhances the effectiveness of the protocol. Maintaining proper hydration becomes especially important, as methylene blue requires adequate fluid levels for optimal distribution and elimination. Supporting cellular health through balanced nutrition and regular physical activity creates an environment that maximizes the benefits of methylene blue.

Protocol development should follow a systematic approach:

- Begin with a baseline health assessment
- Calculate the appropriate starting dose
- Establish consistent administration timing
- Implement supportive lifestyle practices
- Monitor and document response

Quality control remains crucial for the success of the protocol. Using pharmaceutical-grade methylene blue ensures consistent potency and minimizes the risk of contaminants. Proper storage in dark, cool conditions helps maintain the compound's stability and effectiveness over time.

Regular assessment and adjustment of your protocol ensures optimal outcomes. Key monitoring parameters include:

- Energy levels and cognitive function
- Sleep quality and patterns
- Physical performance metrics
- Side effects or adverse reactions[121]
- Overall well-being indicators

The development of a successful protocol requires patience and careful attention to detail. While some individuals may experience benefits quickly, others may need time to determine their optimal dosage and timing. This variability underscores the importance of maintaining detailed records and making systematic adjustments based on observed responses.

Practical implementation strategies should focus on consistency and gradual progression. Starting with a conservative dose allows for proper assessment of individual response while minimizing the risk of adverse effects. As tolerance and comfort develop, careful adjustments can be made to optimize benefits while maintaining safety and security.

A comprehensive protocol summary should include:

- Calculated daily dose based on body weight
- Specific administration timing
- Hydration requirements
- Contraindication awareness
- Monitoring parameters
- Adjustment guidelines

By following these guidelines while respecting individual variations, you can develop a personalized protocol that maximizes the therapeutic potential of methylene blue while maintaining safety and effectiveness. Remember that protocol development is an iterative process that may require adjustment over time as your needs and responses change.

In optimizing the therapeutic potential of methylene blue, we've explored the critical role that lifestyle integration and environmental factors play in maximizing benefits while maintaining safety. From exercise timing and nutritional synergies to sleep optimization and stress management, each component contributes to a comprehensive framework for success.

The process of integrating methylene blue into your daily routine requires careful consideration of multiple factors. We've examined how proper exercise timing can enhance performance and recovery, while strategic nutritional combinations create powerful synergies that amplify therapeutic outcomes. Sleep optimization emerged as a crucial element, highlighting how proper timing of methylene blue administration can support both daytime performance and nighttime recovery.

Stress management and mindfulness practices provide another layer of optimization, working synergistically with methylene blue's cellular-enhancing properties to promote resilience and emotional balance. The importance of aligning with the circadian rhythm cannot be overstated, as it lays the foundation for optimal cellular function and therapeutic response.

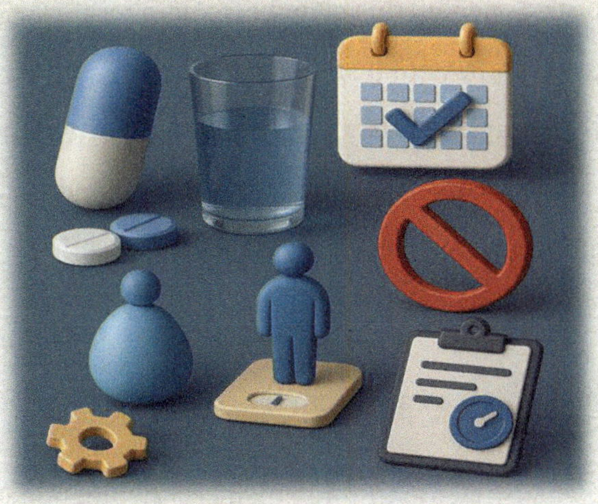

Hydration and detoxification support proved essential for maximizing the effectiveness of methylene blue while ensuring the proper elimination of metabolic byproducts. The careful consideration of environmental factors and exposure optimization highlighted how external conditions can significantly impact therapeutic outcomes.

Perhaps most importantly, we've explored the creation of personalized protocols that respect individual variation while maintaining core therapeutic principles. This personalized approach, combined with careful attention to supplement stacking guidelines, allows for optimal results while minimizing potential risks.

As we conclude this chapter, remember that success with methylene blue therapy relies not just on proper dosing, but on the thoughtful integration of multiple lifestyle factors. By implementing these strategies systematically and monitoring individual response, you can create an environment where methylene blue's cellular-enhancing properties can truly flourish.

The key takeaways from this chapter include:

- Strategic timing enhances therapeutic outcomes
- Lifestyle integration supports optimal results
- Individual response guides protocol development
- Safety considerations remain paramount
- Consistent monitoring ensures sustained benefits

As you move forward with your methylene blue journey, maintain focus on creating sustainable practices that support long-term success. Remember that optimization is an ongoing process, requiring patience and careful attention to individual response. With proper implementation of the strategies outlined in this chapter, you're well-equipped to maximize methylene blue's therapeutic potential while maintaining safety and effectiveness.

Your personal protocol may evolve as you gain experience and better understand your individual response to methylene blue. Stay committed to the core principles we've discussed while remaining flexible enough to make adjustments based on your unique needs and circumstances. This balanced approach, combined with consistent attention to lifestyle factors, creates the foundation for optimal therapeutic outcomes with methylene blue.

Your voice truly matters.

If the book helped you learn something new, feel more empowered about your health, or simply sparked your curiosity, sharing that experience makes a meaningful difference. Simply scan the QR code.

Thank you so much for your time, your support, and for being part of this wellness journey. 💙

CONCLUSION

We have reached the end of our exploration into methylene blue's extraordinary potential, and it's clear this molecule offers far more than its modest beginnings as a textile dye. Throughout this journey, we've uncovered how it energizes cellular powerhouses, protects brain function, and supports nearly every aspect of human vitality.

This subject is deeply personal to me. Living with Young-Onset Parkinson's Disease has allowed me to witness firsthand how methylene blue can transform health and restore function. Its evidence-based effects enhanced mitochondrial performance, improved cognition, and neuroprotection represent more than data; they offer real hope for anyone determined to reclaim their well-being.

Methylene blue stands apart for its direct action on cellular energy production. Functioning as an alternative electron carrier, it strengthens mitochondrial efficiency and powers the body at its core. This fundamental mechanism drives its wide-ranging benefits, from sharper cognition to greater longevity.

The practical protocols and safety guidelines in this book provide a clear roadmap for safe and effective use. Pay close attention to dosage, storage, and integration with lifestyle habits. Begin gradually, observe your body's response, and adjust with intention.

Research continues to reveal new possibilities for methylene blue, marking the dawn of an exciting era in health optimization. The ten benefits explored here may only scratch the surface of its potential to counter cellular decline and age-related deterioration.

Approach this compound with both curiosity and respect. Its impact depends not only on its chemistry but on the wisdom with which it's used. Let the knowledge you've gained guide your choices and shape your pursuit of optimal health.

May this guide serve as both inspiration and instruction. Whether you're managing a condition or pursuing optimal wellness, methylene blue offers a beacon of possibility, a reminder that the future of health is bright, and, fittingly, brilliantly blue.

Your Voice Truly Matters

Thank you so much for your time, your support, and for being part of this wellness journey. 💙

BIBLIOGRAPHY

References

1 Wikipedia contributors. (2024, February 25). Methylene blue. Wikipedia. https://en.wikipedia.org/wiki/Methylene_blue

2 Schwarcz, J.. (2025, October 23). The Right Chemistry: Methylene blue shakes up the medical world. Montreal Gazette. https://montrealgazcttc.com/opinion/columnists/the-right-chemistry-methylene-blue-shakes-up-the-medical-world

3 Odell J.. (2023, October 15). The Rediscovery of Methylene Blue. Bioregulatory Medicine Institute. https://www.brmi.online/post/the-rediscovery-of-methylene-blue

4 Schwarcz, J.. (2025, April 25). TikTok Is Crazy for Methylene Blue, but Not for the Right Reasons. McGill Office for Science and Society. https://www.mcgill.ca/oss/article/medical-critical-thinking-health-and-nutrition/tiktok-crazy-methylene-blue-not-right-reasons

5 Howland R. H.. (2016, September 1). Methylene Blue: The Long and Winding Road From Stain to Brain: Part 1. PubMed. https://pubmed.ncbi.nlm.nih.gov/27576224/

6 National Institute of Standards and Technology. (2023, December 15). Methylene blue. NIST Chemistry WebBook. https://webbook.nist.gov/cgi/cbook.cgi?ID=61-73-4&Units=SI

7 ChemicalBook. (2025-10-23). Methylene Blue. ChemicalBook. https://www.chemicalbook.com/ChemicalProductPropertyENCB2748858.htm

8 BYJU'S. (2019, April 01). What is Methylene blue (C16H18ClN3S)?. BYJU'S. https://byjus.com/chemistry/methylene-blue/

9 National Center for Biotechnology Information. (2025, September 27). Methylene Blue. PubChem. https://pubchem.ncbi.nlm.nih.gov/compound/Methylene-Blue

10 Taylor & Francis Knowledge Centers. (2023). Methylene blue. Taylor & Francis. https://taylorandfrancis.com/knowledge/Engineeringandtechnology/Chemicalengineering/Methyleneblue/

11 Clifton, J.. (2021, July 19). What is the Purpose of Methylene Blue?. Chemicals.co.uk. https://www.chemicals.co.uk/blog/what-is-methylene-blue

12 APC Pure. (2023, December 31). The Chemical Properties of Methylene Blue. APC Pure. https://apcpure.com/news/the-chemical-properties-of-methylene-blue

13 The Calculated Chemist. (2025, January 11). The Fascinating Molecule: Methylene Blue. The Calculated Chemist. https://thecalculatedchemist.com/blogs/news/the-fascinating-molecule-methylene-blue

14 Hover, S.. (2023, August 9). Methylene Blue: From Textile Dye to Potential Clinical Wonder. PCCA Blog. https://www.pccarx.com/Blog/methylene-blue-from-textile-dye-to-potential-clinical-wonder

15 American Chemical Society. (2025, February 10). Methylene Blue. American Chemical Society Molecule of the Week. https://www.acs.org/molecule-of-the-week/archive/m/methylene-blue.html

16 BASF. (2015, February 5). Pioneering thinker - then and now: Methylene blue. BASF-Magazine Creating Chemistry.

https://www.basf.com/global/en/media/magazine/creatingchemistrystories/2015/pioneer-thinker-then-and-now-methlyene-blue

17 Kings Pharmacy and Compounding Center. (2025, April). What Is Methylene Blue? Exploring Its History and Modern Uses. Kings Pharma. https://kingspharma.com/what-is-methylene-blue-exploring-its-history-and-modern-uses/

18 Ellis, R. R.. (2025, April 29). What Is Methylene Blue?. WebMD. https://www.webmd.com/a-to-z-guides/methylene-blue

19 Goldman L. M.. (2025, April 24). What to know about methylene blue. Harvard Health Publishing. https://www.health.harvard.edu/diseases-and-conditions/what-to-know-about-methylene-blue

20 Bakhshi S., Tawfik D.. (2025, May 03). Methylene Blue for the Aging Brain: Mitochondrial Mechanisms Driving Neuroprotective and Cognitive Benefits. Healthspan. https://gethealthspan.com/science/article/methylene-blue-cognitive-benefits

21 Bistas E., Sanghavi D. K.. (2023, June 26). Methylene Blue. StatPearls. https://www.ncbi.nlm.nih.gov/books/NBK557593/

22 Ginimuge P. R.. (2010, October). Methylene Blue: Revisited. Journal of Anaesthesiology, Clinical Pharmacology. https://pmc.ncbi.nlm.nih.gov/articles/PMC3087269/

23 U.S. Food and Drug Administration. (2011, July 26). FDA Drug Safety Communication: Serious CNS reactions possible when methylene blue is given to patients taking certain psychiatric medications. FDA.gov. https://www.fda.gov/drugs/drug-safety-and-availability/fda-drug-safety-communication-serious-cns-reactions-possible-when-methylene-blue-given-patients

24 DrugBank. (2025, October 21). Methylene blue. DrugBank. https://go.drugbank.com/drugs/DB09241

25 Taylor, S.. (2025, September 26). Antiparasitic Agents and Emerging Data on Their Utility as a Cancer Treatment. Fagron Academy. https://www.fagronacademy.us/blog/methylene-blue-understanding-drug-interactions

26 Quaranta, M.. (2023, August 19). Unraveling the Science: Methylene Blue Metabolism in the Human Body. Welltopia Rx. https://welltopiarx.com/unraveling-the-science-methylene-blue-metabolism-in-the-human-body/

27 Cuffari, B.. (2025, March 05). Potential Health Benefits of Methylene Blue. News-Medical.net. https://www.news-medical.net/health/Potential-Health-Benefits-of-Methylene-Blue.aspx

28 Bužga M.. (2022, August 30). Methylene blue: a controversial diagnostic acid and medication?. PMC - US National Library of Medicine. https://pmc.ncbi.nlm.nih.gov/articles/PMC9618115/

29 Locke M.. (2015, June). Methylene Blue and the Risk of Serotonin Toxicity. Anesthesia Patient Safety Foundation. https://www.apsf.org/article/methylene-blue-and-the-risk-of-serotonin-toxicity/

30 Lumistry. (2025, August 13). The Rise of Methylene Blue: What Community Pharmacists Should Know. Lumistry. https://lumistry.com/blog/methylene-blue/

31 Hover, S.. (2023, November). Methylene Blue 15mg capsules. Contigo Compounding. https://contigocompounding.com/methylene-blue/

32 R&D World Staff. (2025, February 6). Methylene blue goes viral—but what is the R&D backstory on this 150-year-old dye?. R&D World. https://www.rdworldonline.com/methylene-blue-goes-viral-but-what-is-the-rd-backstory-on-this-150-year-old-dye/

33 Methylene Blue. (2025, April). History of Methylene Blue. Methylene Blue South Africa. https://methylene-blue.co.za/history/

34 Philly Wellness Center. (2025, February 18). Methylene Blue: Applications, Benefits, and Risks. Philly Wellness Center. https://phillywellnesscenter.com/methylene-blue-applications-benefits-and-risks/

35 The University of Waikato. (2011, July 20). Mitochondria – cell powerhouses. Science Learning Hub. https://www.sciencelearn.org.nz/resources/1839-mitochondria-cell-powerhouses

36 Enzo Life Sciences. (2023, February 06). What is the role of mitochondria in cellular metabolism and bioenergetics?. Enzo.com.https://www.enzo.com/note/what-is-the-role-of-mitochondria-in-cellular-metabolism-and-bioenergetics/

37 Casanova A., Wevers A., Navarro-Ledesma S., Pruimboom L.. (2023, April 25). Mitochondria: It is all about energy. Frontiers in Physiology. https://pmc.ncbi.nlm.nih.gov/articles/PMC10167337/

38 National Human Genome Research Institute. (2025, October 24). Mitochondria. National Human Genome Research Institute. https://www.genome.gov/genetics-glossary/Mitochondria

39 Bell, A.. (2023, March 14). Mitochondria Function, Form and Food.UCLA David Geffen School of Medicine. https://medschool.ucla.edu/news-article/mitochondria-function-form-and-food

40 Nature Education. (2014). Mitochondria. Nature Scitable. https://www.nature.com/scitable/topicpage/mitochondria-14053590/

41 Pfizer Inc.. (2023, October 15). Why Mitochondria Is The Organelle Of The Moment. Pfizer. https://www.pfizer.com/news/articles/whymitochondriaistheorganelleofthe_moment

42 Khan Academy. (2025). Chloroplasts and Mitochondria. Khan Academy. https://www.khanacademy.org/science/ap-biology/cell-structure-and-function/cell-compartmentalization-and-its-origins/a/chloroplasts-and-mitochondria

43 Cleveland Clinic Medical Team. (2023, May 09). Mitochondrial Diseases. Cleveland Clinic. https://my.clevelandclinic.org/health/diseases/15612-mitochondrial-diseases

44 Gonzalez-Lima F., Auchter A.. (2015, May 12). Protection against neurodegeneration with low-dose methylene blue and near-infrared light. Frontiers in Cellular Neuroscience. https://pmc.ncbi.nlm.nih.gov/articles/PMC4428125/

45 Purita, J.. (2025, February 6). Methylene Blue: Revolutionizing Cellular Energy Production. PURFORM Health. https://purformhealth.com/blog/methylene-blue-cellular-energy/

46 Yang S. H.. (2015, November 18). Alternative Mitochondrial Electron Transfer for the Treatment of Neurodegenerative Diseases and Cancers: Methylene Blue Connects the Dots. Progress in Neurobiology. https://pmc.ncbi.nlm.nih.gov/articles/PMC4871783/

47 PatSnap. (2024, July 17). What is the mechanism of Methylene blue?. Synapse. https://synapse.patsnap.com/article/what-is-the-mechanism-of-methylene-blue

48 AgelessRx. (2024). The Science Behind the Blue: How Methylene Blue Works. AgelessRx. https://agelessrx.com/the-science-behind-the-blue-how-methylene-blue-works/

49 Advanced IV Health. (2025, January 28). What Is Methylene Blue Used For? Supporting Mitochondrial Health. Advanced IV Health. https://advancedivhealth.com/blog/what-is-methylene-blue-used-for-supporting-mitochondrial-health

50 Gonzalez-Lima F.. (2015, May 11). Protection against neurodegeneration with low-dose methylene blue and near-infrared light. Frontiers in Cellular Neuroscience. https://www.frontiersin.org/journals/cellular-neuroscience/articles/10.3389/fncel.2015.00179/full

51 Poudel S. B.. (2024, March 25). Targeting mitochondrial dysfunction using methylene blue or mitoquinone to improve skeletal aging. PMC – PubMed Central. https://pmc.ncbi.nlm.nih.gov/articles/PMC11006499/

52 Kings Pharmacy and Compounding Center. (2025, April). The Role of Methylene Blue in Fighting Oxidative Stress and Aging. Kings Pharma. https://kingspharma.com/the-role-of-methylene-blue-in-fighting-oxidative-stress-and-aging/

53 Xue H., Thaivalappil A., Cao K.. (2021, December 1). The Potentials of Methylene Blue as an Anti-Aging Drug. PMC – PubMed Central. https://pmc.ncbi.nlm.nih.gov/articles/PMC8699482/

54 Xiong Z. M. et al. (2017, May 30). Anti-Aging Potentials of Methylene Blue for Human Skin Longevity. Scientific Reports. https://www.nature.com/articles/s41598-017-02419-3

55 Poteet E.. (2012, October 31). Neuroprotective Actions of Methylene Blue and Its Derivatives. PLOS ONE. https://journals.plos.org/plosone/article?id=10.1371%2Fjournal.pone.0048279

56 National Library of Medicine. (2022, October 1). Methylene blue as a neuroprotective agent: mechanisms of action. PubMed. https://pubmed.ncbi.nlm.nih.gov/36180986/

57 St. Onge, A.. (2024, May 28). Exploring Low-Dose Oral Methylene Blue for Mitochondrial Support. Integrative Practitioner. https://www.integrativepractitioner.com/featured/exploring-low-dose-oral-methylene-blue-for-mitochondrial-support/

58 Renoja Research Team. (2025, March). Methylene Blue and Its Impact on Mitochondrial Function: A Deep Dive. Renoja. https://renoja.com/methylene-blue-and-its-impact-on-mitochondrial-function-a-deep-dive/

59 Dakota Pharmacy. (2025, August 7). Methylene Blue Dosing Explained: Benefits, Risks, and What Science Says. DakotaRx. https://dakotarx.com/methylene-blue-dosing-explained-benefits-risks-and-what-science-says

60 AgelessRx. (2023, December 15). Methylene Blue Dosing: Debunking Misconceptions About Safety. AgelessRx. https://agelessrx.com/methylene-blue-dosing-debunking-misconceptions-about-safety/

61 Healing Dose Compounding Pharmacy. (2023, March 14). Methylene Blue & Improving Mitochondrial Function – Michigan Compounding Pharmacy. HDRx. https://www.hdrx.com/methylene-blue-improving-mitochondrial-function/

62 NatureMed Integrative Medicine. (2025, January 01). Methylene Blue Benefits in Longevity Medicine. NatureMed Clinic. https://www.naturemedclinic.com/methylene-blue-benefits-in-longevity-medicine/

63 Tucker D., Lu Y., Zhang Q.. (2017, August 24). From Mitochondrial Function to Neuroprotection - An Emerging Role for Methylene Blue. PMC - National Library of Medicine. https://pmc.ncbi.nlm.nih.gov/articles/PMC5826781/

64 Dempsey, T.. (2023, November). What Is Methylene Blue? A Look At Its Surprising Health Benefits. Dr. Tania Dempsey. https://drtaniadempsey.com/what-is-methylene-blue-a-look-at-its-surprising-health-benefits/

65 Elite NP. (2025, August 25). Methylene Blue: Clinical Applications for Functional Medicine Success. Elite NP. https://elitenp.com/methylene-blue-clinical-applications-for-functional-medicine-success/

66 NADclinic. (2025, May 9). Beat Chronic Fatigue With Methylene Blue. NADclinic. https://nadclinic.com/beat-chronic-fatigue-with-methylene-blue/

67 Johnson, C.. (2023, December 26). A Methylene Blue Boost? Could a Blue Dye Help with ME/CFS, Long COVID and Fibromyalgia?. Health Rising. https://www.healthrising.org/blog/2023/12/26/methylene-blue-chronic-fatigue-syndrome-long-covid-fibromyalgia/

68 417 Integrative Medicine. (2025, July 1). Here's What to Know About Methylene Blue for Energy and Focus. 417 Integrative Medicine. https://www.417integrativemedicine.com/articles/heres-what-to-know-about-methylene-blue-for-energy-and-focus

69 National Library of Medicine. (2014, August 11). Methylene blue attenuates cognitive deficits caused by chronic cerebral hypoperfusion in rats. PubMed. https://pubmed.ncbi.nlm.nih.gov/25079810/

70 Rojas J. C., Bruchey A. K., Gonzalez-Lima F.. (2011, November 3). Neurometabolic mechanisms for memory enhancement and neuroprotection of methylene blue. Progress in Neurobiology. https://pmc.ncbi.nlm.nih.gov/articles/PMC3265679/

71 RSNA Media Relations. (2016, June 28). Methylene Blue Shows Promise for Improving Short-Term Memory. Radiological Society of North America. https://www.rsna.org/media/press/i/1888

72 BioLight. (2024, March 29). Antimicrobial Properties of Methylene Blue: Fighting Infections Effectively. BioLight Shop. https://www.biolight.shop/blogs/methylene-blue/antimicrobial-properties-of-methylene-blue-fighting-infections-effectively

73 Akina Pharmacy. (2024, June). Methylene Blue: A Closer Look. Akina Pharmacy. https://akinapharmacy.com/methyleneblue/

74 National Library of Medicine. (2022, December 28). Methylene blue has antibacterial effects that might interfere with microbial culture in vitro. PubMed. https://pubmed.ncbi.nlm.nih.gov/36577990/

75 Songsantiphap C., Vanichanan J., Chatsuwan T., Asawanonda P., Boontaveeyuwat E.. (2022, July 1). Methylene Blue–Mediated Antimicrobial Photodynamic Therapy Against Clinical Isolates of Extensively Drug Resistant Gram-Negative Bacteria Causing Nosocomial Infections in Thailand, An In Vitro Study. Frontiers in Cellular and Infection Microbiology. https://pmc.ncbi.nlm.nih.gov/articles/PMC9283779/

76 Windsor W. J.. (2022, March 8). Methylene Blue: The Little-Known Disinfectant. American Society for Microbiology. https://asm.org/articles/2022/march/methylene-blue-the-little-known-disinfectant

77 Relive Health. (2025, September 19). Methylene Blue: Everything You Need to Know About This Remarkable Compound. Relive Health. https://relivehealth.com/iv-vitamin-therapy/methylene-blue-everything-you-need-to-know-about-this-remarkable-compound/

78 Atamna H.. (2015, September 10). Combined activation of the energy and cellular-defense pathways may explain the potent anti-senescence activity of methylene blue. Redox Biology. https://pmc.ncbi.nlm.nih.gov/articles/PMC4588422/

79 CORR Pasadena. (2023, December 15). Methylene Blue: Neurological Benefits & Brain Health Support. CORR Heal. https://corrheal.com/blog/methylene-blue-neurological-benef/

80 Zhao C-C, Zhai Y-J, Hu Z-J, Huo Y, Li Z-Q, Zhu G-J. (2022, September 25). Efficacy and safety of methylene blue in patients with vasodilatory shock: A systematic review and meta-analysis. Frontiers in Medicine. https://www.frontiersin.org/journals/medicine/articles/10.3389/fmed.2022.950596/full

81 Fernandes Junior, H. J.. (2024, November 11). Cardiotoxic and Cardioprotective Effects of Methylene Blue in the Animal Model of Cardiac Ischemia and Reperfusion. PMC - US National Library of Medicine. https://pmc.ncbi.nlm.nih.gov/articles/PMC11591808/

82 iPerfusion. (2025, February 05). The Mystery of Methylene Blue and Its Role in Managing Post-Cardiac Surgery Vasoplegic Shock. iPerfusion. https://iperfusion.org/the-mystery-of-

methylene-blue-and-its-role-in-managing-post-cardiac-surgery-vasoplegic-shock/

83 National Library of Medicine. (2019, June 1). Methylene Blue: The Long and Winding Road From Stain to Brain. PubMed. https://pubmed.ncbi.nlm.nih.gov/31144270/

84 AMFM Treatment. (2025, July). What is Methylene Blue & Does It Help with Depression?. AMFM Treatment. https://amfmtreatment.com/what-we-treat/depression/methylene-blue-depression/

85 LaFountain R.. (2024, April 30). What's the Optimal Dose of Methylene Blue for Depression?. Healthspan. https://gethealthspan.com/science/article/methylene-blue-dose-for-depression

86 AgelessRx. (2023). Methylene Blue for Energy & Longevity: A Deep Dive. AgelessRx. https://agelessrx.com/methylene-blue-for-energy-longevity-a-deep-dive/

87 Gowing Life. (2024, August 5). The Curious Case Of Methylene Blue, A Dye That Might Slow Ageing. Gowing Life. https://www.gowinglife.com/the-curious-case-of-methylene-blue-a-dye-that-might-slow-ageing/

88 Dean, G.. (2024, April 30). Biohacker Gary Brecka on the Anti-Aging Capabilities of Methylene Blue. NAD.com. https://www.nad.com/news/biohacker-gary-brecka-on-the-anti-aging-capabilities-of-methylene-blue

89 Xiong Z. M.. (2017, May 24). Methylene blue reduces skin fibrosis by improving redox homeostasis. PubMed. https://pubmed.ncbi.nlm.nih.gov/28559565/

90 Kayabaşı Y., Erbaş O.. (2023). Methylene blue and its importance in medicine. Journal of Medical Developments, Breakthroughs and Updates. https://www.journalmeddbu.com/full-text/213

91 National Library of Medicine. (2017, July 28). Dichotomic effects of methylene blue on mitochondrial respiratory function and ROS production in diabetic and nondiabetic rat heart mitochondria. PubMed. https://pubmed.ncbi.nlm.nih.gov/28738167/

92 Permana, M. D.. (2023, January 23). A Simple Methods for Determination of Methylene Blue using Smartphone-Based as Digital Image Colorimetry. Thammasat International Science and Technology Journal. https://tis.wu.ac.th/index.php/tis/article/download/5149/532

93 American Public Health Association. (2023). Standard Methods: 4500-S2- D: Sulfide by Methylene Blue. National Environmental Methods Index. https://www.nemi.gov/methods/method_summary/7418/

94 BRC HEALTHCARE. (2024, August 13). Methylene Blue Dosage Chart: Accurate Guidelines for Safe Administration. BRC Recovery. https://brcrecovery.com/blogs/methylene-blue-dosage-chart/

95 Chase, N.. (2025, July 10). Methylene Blue Dosage Chart. Era Organics. https://www.eraorganics.com/blogs/beauty-guide/methylene-blue-dosage

96 Hakim, R. C.. (2025, January 2). Methylene Blue Dosage. GoodRx. https://www.goodrx.com/methylene-blue/dosage

97 Eden Health. (2025, June 24). Methylene Blue Safety: Key Risks and Best Practices. Eden Health. https://www.tryeden.com/post/methylene-blue-safety

98 Kings Pharma. (2025, March). How Does Methylene Blue Interact with Other Medications?. Kings Pharma. https://kingspharma.com/how-does-methylene-blue-interact-with-other-medications/

99. Khan, S.. (2024). Methylene Blue. RxList. https://www.rxlist.com/methylene_blue/generic-drug.htm

100 Merative. (2025, October 01). Methylene Blue (Intravenous Route) – Side Effects & Uses. Mayo Clinic. https://www.mayoclinic.org/drugs-supplements/methylene-blue-intravenous-route/description/drg-20064695

101 Gillman P. K.. (2010, February). CNS toxicity involving methylene blue: the exemplar for understanding and predicting drug interactions that precipitate serotonin toxicity. PubMed. https://pubmed.ncbi.nlm.nih.gov/20142303/

102 MedicineNet. (2023, December 31). METHYLENE BLUE - ORAL. MedicineNet.com. https://www.medicinenet.com/methylene_blue-oral/article.htm

103 Innovating Science. (2023, November 14). Methylene Blue Solution, 1%, Aqueous, 100 mL. CalPacLab. https://www.calpaclab.com/methylene-blue-solution-1-percent-aqueous-100ml-innovating-science/ad-mm0440-100ml

104 Burkhardt, M. R., Cinotto, P. J., Frahm, G. W., Woodworth, M. T., & Pritt, J. W.. (1995). Methods of analysis by the U.S. Geological Survey National Water Quality Laboratory-Determination of methylene blue active substances by

spectrophotometry. U.S. Geological Survey. https://pubs.usgs.gov/publication/ofr95189

105 Lee S. E.. (2024, June 15). Evaluation of Methylene Blue Migration from Time—Temperature Indicators Using LC-MS/MS. PMC – PubMed Central. https://pmc.ncbi.nlm.nih.gov/articles/PMC11202443/

106 HEALR. (2024, January 15). Methylene Blue Safety: Why Purity Testing Matters. HEALR Blog. https://drinkhealr.com/blogs/healr-blu3-studies/methylene-blue-safety-why-purity-testing-matters

107 Torres, M. R.. (2025, July 23). Methylene Blue in Tactical Medicine: A Guide for Cops, Paramedics, and Prepared Civilians. Tactical Medicine. https://tactical-medicine.com/blogs/news/methylene-blue-in-tactical-medicine-a-guide-for-cops-paramedics-and-prepared-civilians

108 LabChem, Inc.. (2019, August 15). Methylene Blue Safety Data Sheet. SafeSchools SDS. https://e2ccb-ny.newlook.safeschoolssds.com/document/repo/4ae6ad6f-1650-4b5f-a3f9-9e69b04c8e07

109 Xue S., Li L., Liu Z. et al.. (2025, March 01). Predicting responsiveness to fixed-dose methylene blue in adult patients with septic shock using interpretable machine learning: a retrospective study. Scientific Reports. https://www.nature.com/articles/s41598-025-89934-w

110 Eden Medical Team. (2025, June 24). Methylene Blue Dosage: Guidelines for Safe & Effective Use. Eden. https://www.tryeden.com/post/methylene-blue-dosage

111 Justice LA Now. (2021, January 01). How To Take Methylene Blue Tincture Safely and Clearly. Justice LA Now. https://justicelanow.org/art/howtotakemethylenebluetincturesafelyandclearly.html

112 BioLight. (2024, March 30). How Methylene Blue Can Improve Your Workout Routine. BioLight Shop. https://www.biolight.shop/blogs/methylene-blue/how-methylene-blue-can-improve-your-workout-routine

113 Vorhauer, L.. (2024, March 20). Methylene Blue for Endurance: What the Science Says. Troscriptions. https://troscriptions.com/blogs/main/methylene-blue-for-endurance

114 Murphy, J.. (2025, September 2). Unlocking the Power of Methylene Blue: A Revolutionary Wellness Treatment. The IV Hub Wellness. https://theivhubwellness.com/unlocking-the-power-of-methylene-blue-a-revolutionary-wellness-treatment/

115 RELIVE Health. (2025, August 22). The Role of Methylene Blue in Anti-Aging Medicine: Why It's Getting Attention. RELIVE Health. https://relivehealth.com/anti-aging/nad-and-5-amino-1mq-synergy-in-therapy-2/

116 Frederick, M.. (2024, February 09). Methylene Blue and Intermittent Fasting: A Synergistic Approach to Health and Longevity. NOBIESSE. https://nobiesse.com/blogs/knowledge-center/methylene-blue-and-intermittent-fasting-a-synergistic-approach-to-health-and-longevity

117 Bubs Naturals. (2025, August 29). Can You Take Methylene Blue with Vitamin C? Exploring the Synergistic Benefits. Bubs Naturals. https://www.bubsnaturals.com/blogs/all-about-vitamin-c/can-you-take-methylene-blue-with-vitamin-c-exploring-the-synergistic-benefits

118 Mobile Meraki. (2025, March 28). Methylene Blue: The Biohacking Trend & Its Connection to Longevity and Wellness. Meraki Integrative. https://www.merakiintegrative.com/methylene-blue

119 AgelessRx. (2024, January 15). Methylene Blue vs. Traditional Nootropics: What You Need to Know. AgelessRx. https://agelessrx.com/methylene-blue-vs-traditional-nootropics-what-you-need-to-know/

120 Philipose, A.. (2025, June 9). The Benefits of Methylene Blue Infusion Therapy in Oklahoma City. Venturis Clinic. https://venturisclinic.com/regenerative-medicine-blog/the-benefits-of-methylene-blue-infusion-therapy-in-oklahoma-city/

121 Piazza Center. (2024, January 15). 5 Benefits of Methylene Blue—And Other Unexpected Power Tools Dr. Piazza Recommends. The Piazza Center. https://www.thepiazzacenter.com/blog/5-benefits-of-methylene-blue-and-other-unexpected-power-tools-dr-piazza-recommend/

122 Ringside Health. (2025, May 15). The Science Behind Methylene Blue: A Game-Changer in Functional Medicine. Ringside Health. https://www.ringsidehealth.com/post/the-science-behind-methylene-blue-a-game-changer-in-functional-medicine

123 Liester M. B.. (2024, October 8). Red Light Therapy and Methylene Blue May Promote Brain Health. Psychology Today. https://www.psychologytoday.com/us/blog/the-leading-edge/202409/red-light-therapy-and-methylene-blue-may-promote-brain-health

124 Fustin, J. M., Ye, S., Rakers, C. et al.. (2020, May 06). Methylation deficiency disrupts biological rhythms from bacteria to humans. Nature Communications Biology. https://www.nature.com/articles/s42003-020-0942-0

125 Race K., Jolly S., Bakhshi S.. (2024, September 14). Circadian Rhythm Synchronization as a Strategy for Enhancing Healthspan and Preventing Metabolic Disorders. Healthspan. https://gethealthspan.com/science/article/circadian-rhythm-healthspan-metabolic-optimization

126 Fang M. Z.. (2010, April 27). Methylselenocysteine Resets the Rhythmic Expression of Circadian and Growth Regulatory Genes Disrupted by Nitrosomethylurea in vivo. PMC - National Center for Biotechnology Information. https://pmc.ncbi.nlm.nih.gov/articles/PMC2865563/

127 Relive Health. (2025, May 13). How Methylene Blue Supports Cognitive Health. Relive Health. https://relivehealth.com/iv-vitamin-therapy/how-methylene-blue-supports-cognitive-health/

128 Dauchy R. T.. (2018, August). Effect of Daytime Blue-enriched LED Light on the Nighttime Circadian Melatonin Inhibition of Hepatoma 7288CTC Warburg Effect and Progression. PMC - US National Library of Medicine. https://pmc.ncbi.nlm.nih.gov/articles/PMC6103418/

129 IV Boost. (2025, March 28). Methylene Blue IV Drips – Benefits and FAQs. IV Boost UK. https://ivboost.uk/methylene-blue-iv-drips-benefits-and-faqs/

130 Axon Integrative Health. (2023, June 01). Unlocking Neuro Protection and Enhancements: The Power of Methylene Blue IV Therapy. Axon Integrative Health. https://axonintegrativehealth.com/iv-packages/unlocking-neuro-protection-and-enhancements-the-power-of-methylene-blue-iv-therapy/

131 IV Elements. (2023, May 01). At-Home Methylene Blue IV Therapy. IVElements.net. https://ivelements.net/methyl-blue-iv

132 Bellava Aesthetics. (2025, June). Methylene Blue IV Therapy and Brain Power: Cognitive Enhancement Backed by Science. Bellava Aesthetics. https://bellavaaesthetics.com/methylene-blue-iv-therapy-and-brain-power-cognitive-enhancement-backed-by-science/

133 Mind Mend. (2025, February 13). Stacking Methylene Blue: What Works and What to Avoid. Mind Mend. https://www.mindmend.co/stacking-methylene-blue-what-works-and-what-to-avoid/

134 Cole, W.. (2024, January). What Are The Benefits + Uses Of Methylene Blue?. Dr. Will Cole. https://drwillcole.com/how-to-use-methylene-blue/

135 Defy Medical. (2025, June). What Supplements to Take with Methylene Blue. Defy Medical. https://www.defymedical.com/blog/what-supplements-to-take-with-methylene-blue/

136 Whole Health Glebe. (2023, October 15). Why Compounded Methylene Blue Might Be the Brain Boost You've Been Looking For. Whole Health Glebe. https://wholehealthglebe.com/uncategorized/why-compounded-methylene-blue-might-be-the-brain-boost-youve-been-looking-for/

137 Liu J.. (2021, September 23). Optimization of Decoloration Conditions of Methylene Blue Wastewater by Penicillium P1. PMC – National Library of Medicine. https://pmc.ncbi.nlm.nih.gov/articles/PMC8758838/

138 Maniyam M. N., Hari M.. (2021, July 05). Optimization of culture conditions for improved green biodecolourization of methylene blue by Rhodococcus pyridinivorans strain UCC 0003. BioTechnologia. https://www.biotechnologia-

journal.org/Optimization-of-culture-conditions-for-improved-green-biodecolourization-of-methylene,133622,0,2.html

Made in the USA
Monee, IL
03 November 2026

67384804R00144